# Natural Pregnancy A–Z

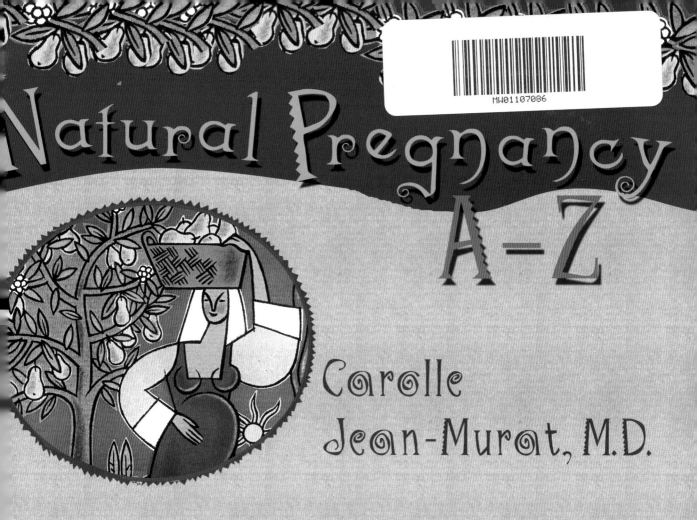

Carolle
Jean-Murat, M.D.

Hay House, Inc.
Carlsbad, California • Sydney, Australia

LIFE Styles

Published and distributed in the United States by:
Hay House, Inc., P.O. Box 5100, Carlsbad, CA 92018-5100 • (800) 654-5126 • (800) 650-5115 (fax)

*Editorial:* Jill Kramer     *Cover Design:* Christy Salinas     *Interior Design:* Jenny Richards
*Illustrations:* Jean-Manuel Duvivier

LIBRARY OF CONGRESS CATALOGING-IN-PUBLICATION DATA

Jean-Murat, Carolle.
    Natural pregnancy A-Z / Carolle Jean-Murat.
        p.  cm.
    ISBN 1-56170-709-0
    1. Pregnancy.  2. Natural childbirth. I. Title.
  RG526 .J43 2000
  618'.03--dc21                99-045797

ISBN 1-56170-709-0

03 02 01 00     4 3 2 1
First Printing, April 2000

Printed by Palace Press Hong Kong

# Contents

Contents, cont.'d

# Introduction

Pregnancy is, first of all, a *natural* occurrence in the life of a woman. Women have been doing it for millions of years, and until recently, doing it naturally. While it's comforting to know that you have the benefits of modern medicine at your fingertips, please know that *planning* to get pregnant, *getting* pregnant, and giving birth (if there are no major complications) can still be a happy, natural occasion.

The outcome of a pregnancy depends greatly on your state of health and your lifestyle before you ever become pregnant. Proper preconceptual and prenatal care go hand in hand with having a healthy baby, regardless of your age.

The best way to start the process is to take proper care of yourself even before you try to become pregnant. The fertilized egg (the embryo) draws all its nutrients from the endometrium—the thick, blood-filled lining of the uterus. The embryo implants itself upon the endometrium and begins to develop into a baby ready for birth approximately 40 weeks later. The nutrients supplied by the endometrium come directly from what you put into your own body.

Many birth defects occur during the first two weeks of pregnancy, often at a time when the woman does not know she is pregnant. Birth defects can be hereditary, but they can also be caused by toxic substances, viral infections, nutritional deficiencies, radiation from x-rays, some prescription medicines, drugs, and alcohol. While the mother's health and activities can help to prevent many birth defects, some defects are beyond the mother's, or anyone's, control. If there is a family history of birth defects or inherited disorders, check with your health-care provider about genetic testing before you try to conceive.

Before becoming pregnant, have your dentist take care of any cavities, since the body reroutes minerals used for tooth maintenance to the unborn child. Hopefully, you already have a good relationship with the health-care provider who will care for you while you're pregnant. Discuss your respective views on childbirth to see if they coincide. If you don't agree, it may be appropriate to find another health-care provider. If you have any medical problems, now is the time to get them resolved or under control. *Don't wait until after you become pregnant.*

It is a good idea to be in optimal physical health and within five pounds of your ideal weight before conceiving. You should stop taking all over-the-counter medications, except folic acid found in vitamin B-complex or multivitamin supplements. The U.S. Public Health Service recommends that all women of childbearing age consume at least 0.4 mg of folic acid each day. Taking multivitamin supplements with folic acid during the three months before becoming pregnant has been demonstrated to reduce the risk of neural-tube defects. If you must take prescribed medications, talk to your health-care provider to make sure they are not known to cause birth defects. If necessary, your physician may be able to provide safer alternatives.

Avoid all toxic substances such as alcohol and other drugs; drinking can reduce a woman's chance of getting pregnant. If you smoke, this is a good time to quit. Taking herbs or over-the counter supplements, which many people consider harmless, can be risky. For example, high dosages of St. John's wort, ginkgo biloba, and echinacea have been shown to have an adverse effect on fertilization.

Make sure you are vaccinated against or are immune to Rubella (German measles). If a woman contracts Rubella during pregnancy, especially during the first three months, it could cause serious birth defects. Because of the potential risk to the developing fetus, vaccines should be administered as part of the pre-conception evaluation.

If you are taking the Pill, switch to a barrier method of birth control (such as condoms together with foam) for at least three cycles before trying to become pregnant. It may take up to six to eight weeks for some women who have been on the Pill to begin having a regular cycle. Once your cycle becomes regular, it will be much easier to determine when you become pregnant, and to calculate your due date.

The father shares an important role in the outcome of a healthy baby. Just like the female egg, sperm are vulnerable to genetic and environmental influences, and the seminal fluid may contain harmful materials. If the father abuses drugs or alcohol, if he smokes tobacco, or if he is exposed to toxic agents in the environment, he can negatively affect the health of his offspring. Many studies have demonstrated a direct correla-

tion between industrial compounds and possible risks to the baby. Some studies have found that the pregnant wives of men who are occupationally exposed to materials such as latex, plastics, benzene, and toluene, have an increased risk of spontaneous abortion (miscarriage).

A study in British Columbia recently revealed that children born of fathers employed as firemen had a higher risk of congenital heart defects, possibly due to the toxic chemicals the men were exposed to in the line of duty. Prospective fathers should follow the same advice given to women who are trying to become pregnant: Do not drink; use drugs; or smoke before, during, or after pregnancy; and do not become exposed to toxic substances in the environment.

The healthy development of children, and the family as a whole, is enhanced by a man who is supportive of his partner and promotes healthful habits and a stable home environment.

Many women are used to being in charge of their lives, planning everything and working hard to succeed. Many women go to college, achieve postgraduate degrees, have successful careers, and postpone pregnancy for years. One day they decide to get pregnant and want it to happen NOW.

Sorry, it does not work that way. Only about one in four women will conceive after the first try; it can take an average of eight months for 80 percent of women who are having regular, unprotected intercourse two or three times a week to get pregnant. So, please do not come running into my medical office wondering what is wrong with you! In a rare case, one of my patients had four children, all conceived exactly two years apart. Your body will let it happen when it is ready.

Have fun with your partner while trying to get pregnant, but do not make it a chore. If your next period comes, do not view this as the end of the world. Be patient. My personal opinion is that women who are stressed about conceiving may indeed delay conception. You've probably heard the occasional story of the couple told they were infertile who decided to adopt a child, only to become pregnant shortly after the adoption.

During your pregnancy, follow the advice of your health-care provider. Keep your appointments as scheduled, and have the tests that are recommended. When it comes to getting the tests for birth defects—alpha-feto-protein (AFP), chorionic villus sampling (CVS), and amniocentesis—remember that whether or not you have them done is a personal choice. Some women want to know, at any cost, if their baby will be born healthy; they often choose to terminate any pregnancy upon learning that their baby has a birth defect. Yet, many other women believe that a child is a gift from God and would welcome a baby whether or not there are abnormalities. These women decline any such testing.

Birthing used to be considered a natural event—it took place in the home and was overseen by midwives, or "sage femmes." My first experience with a home birth was at the age of 11 when I accompanied my mother, a sage-femme, to a delivery in rural Haiti. Later on, during my year of community medicine in rural Mexico, more than 25 deliveries were done in the home, often with no running water or electricity available. In North America, this trend underwent a dramatic shift in the beginning of the 20th century, when births moved to hospitals and were attended by male doctors. Today, births rarely ever occur at home; in fact, it is not recommended if there are any risk factors that may result in complications during labor or delivery. If you decide on a home birth, you should carefully investigate the reputation of your birth attendant and learn what arrangements have been made in case of an emergency.

Most deliveries occur without complications, but when problems arise, it can be life threatening for both mother and baby. Most complications can be taken care of at the hospital.

Wherever you choose to give birth, it is a good idea to have a "birth plan." Convey your wishes to the people who are taking care of you, and be willing to accept intervention when advised. Most hospitals allow partner to be present, even during a cesarean section (C-section).

During labor, at a hospital facility you will be cared for by the resident doctor on duty, or a nurse midwife, the nursing staff, and, on occasion, a medical student. These people remain in constant contact with your health-care provider and notify him or her of any complications and when delivery is imminent.

During the labor process, you can sip water or juice. You do not want to have a full stomach. One of the causes of maternal death is aspiration during general anesthesia. Vomiting and retching is common during the late stages of labor.

9

With managed care, you may find that when you become pregnant you are no longer able to see the health-care provider with whom you have built a trusting relationship over the years. The idea of a solo practitioner who cares for you throughout your entire pregnancy and delivery is practically extinct. Most obstetricians are part of large practices who share calls for hospital deliveries. If you have been followed by a nurse practitioner at a clinic, you will probably be delivered by someone else at the hospital.

If you do not have a satisfactory relationship with your health-care provider, pay some consideration to finding a new provider, regardless of how far you are into the pregnancy. It is natural to trust yourself. It is true that *your health lies in your hands*, and you should enter into a relationship with your health-care provider where you are allowed to take part in the decision making. You must admit that you do not have the appropriate training and experience required to decide the best course to follow if an emergency arises, and you need to trust your health-care provider.

Remember, your pregnancy is an opportunity to learn about the effects of tension, stress, eating, and other habits on your health and state of mind—lessons that will prove helpful for the rest of your life.

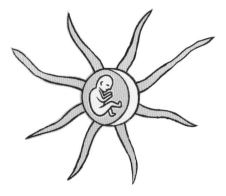

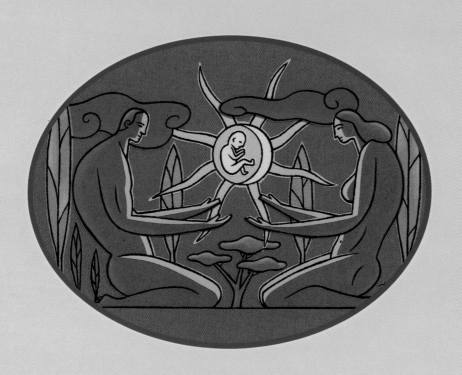

A

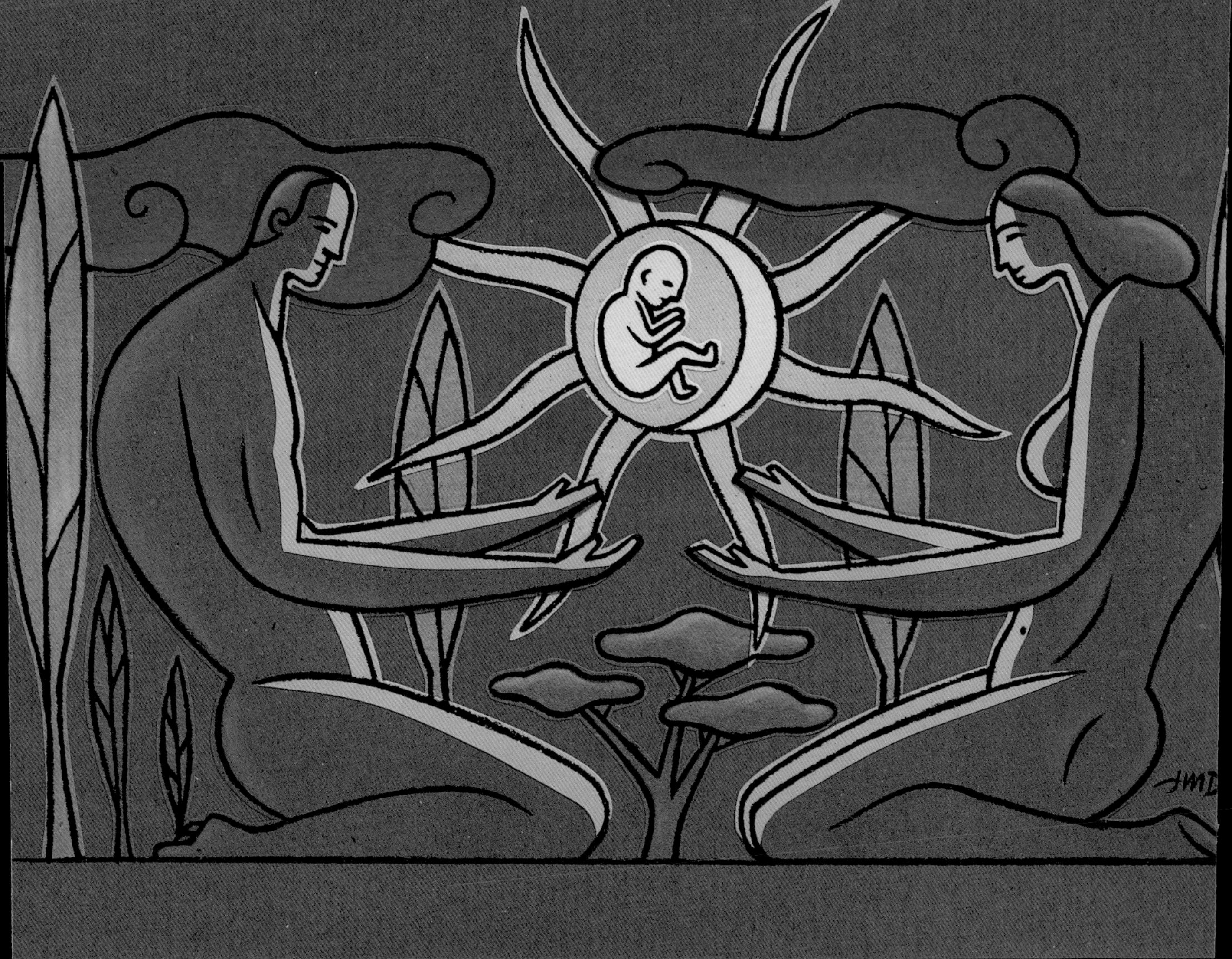

# The A-Z List

## Abortion

To the lay person, an abortion is the act of voluntarily terminating a pregnancy. The decision to terminate a pregnancy is a woman's personal choice. The type of abortion performed depends upon the length of the pregnancy. During the first trimester (the first 12 weeks after the last menstrual period), the typical procedure is vacuum aspiration, in which a suction instrument removes the embryo or fetus and the placenta. RU 486, an abortion-inducing pill, can also be used during the first six weeks after the last menstrual period. This treatment is not generally available in the United States; but is available in France, the United Kingdom, and other countries. During the second trimester, several procedures are used. If the pregnancy is 13 to 16 weeks, dilation and evacuation (similar to vacuum aspiration) can be performed. If the pregnancy is 16 to 24 weeks, it is more common to induce labor by injecting fluid—usually saline or prostaglandin hormones—into the amniotic sac. Hysterotomy (an incision into the uterus), and (in extreme cases), hysterectomy, can also be performed.

## Acetaminophen

Acetaminophen (Tylenol) is considered safe for occasional use during pregnancy. Your best bet is to check with your health-care provider first.

## Acupressure

This treatment can be used to relieve pain due to headache and backache caused by pregnancy. Acupressure is based upon the concept of qi (also known as chi), or energy. Finger pressure, instead of needles, is employed at acupuncture points. This treatment can be effective, but results may be less dramatic than acupuncture.

## Acupuncture

Acupuncture is a medical application that has been in use for more than 6,000 years. This treatment can be used to relieve pain due to headache and backache, as well as relieving discomfort due to hemorrhoids during pregnancy.

## Afterbirth

Also called the placenta.

## AIDS

A disease known as "Acquired Immunodeficiency Syndrome," and probably caused by the HIV virus. See *HIV*.

## Alcohol

If you are trying to get pregnant, you should stop drinking alcohol entirely. No amount of alcohol has been determined to be safe for the fetus. The first eight weeks after conception are critical to fetal development. Drinking during pregnancy may cause one or more of the following: facial deformity, low-set ears, heart murmur, mental retardation, and hyperactivity. These abnormalities have become known as Fetal Alcohol Syndrome. However, you do not need to worry about having had an occasional glass of wine or bee prior to learning that you were pregnant.

## Allergies

Due to hormonal changes, allergies may clear up or worsen during pregnancy. Allergy medications, nasal sprays, and shots are usually safe, but you should check with your health-care provider before using any medication.

## Alpha-Feto-Protein (AFP)

During your pregnancy, your health-care provider may want to perform some specific tests. One of these tests is the alpha-feto-protein (AFP), which is used to rule out defects of the unborn baby's nervous system between the 15th and 20th week. If your levels are elevated, this does not necessarily mean that the fetus has a neural tube defect. Your health-care provider may perform a detailed ultrasound evaluation or obtain amniotic fluid via an amniocentesis to re-measure the AFP. In most cases of elevated AFP levels, the babies are normal.

## Amenorrhea

This term refers to the lack of menstrual periods. After stopping the Pill, a small percentage of women will have no periods for as long as three months. Some women who have used Depo-Provera, especially women who used it for many years, may have to wait at least one year before their normal menstrual cycle resumes.

## Amniocentesis

Amniocentesis involves the sampling of fluid from the bag of water that surrounds the baby in order to test the genetic makeup of fetal cells that have been shed into the fluid. It is usually performed between the 15th and 20th week of gestation under ultrasound guidance. This procedure carries a very low risk of fetal loss. Amniocentesis can also be performed near the delivery date to confirm that the lungs of the fetus are mature.

## Amnio-Infusion

When the fetal heart rate suggests that the fetus is in distress due to an umbilical cord compression, a sterile, balanced saline solution can be infused into the uterine cavity to try to relieve the pressure on the umbilical cord.

## Amniotic Fluid

This fluid is contained in the bag of water surrounding the baby. Waste products and cells from the fetus are also discarded into the fluid.

## Amniotic Sac

Also known as the "bag of water," or amniotic membranes; these are thin membranes filled with amniotic fluid containing the fetus. Stripping of the amniotic membranes is commonly done to induce labor. Also see *Water Breaks.*

## Amniotomy

This is the procedure where the "bag of water" is artificially ruptured during labor. It usually ruptures naturally toward the end of the first stage of labor, and sometimes before labor. In certain cases, it must be artificially ruptured using a tool not unlike a crochet hook. Amniotomy may be used to induce labor.

## Analgesic

During labor, pain can be relieved by injecting a narcotic analgesic into a muscle or via an intravenous line. Side effects in the mother may include drowsiness and a decreased ability to concentrate. In the newborn baby, reflexes and breathing are slowed down. For this reason, an analgesic is given during early labor and avoided just before delivery.

## Anemia

During pregnancy, your blood volume doubles, often reducing your iron levels. During your first prenatal visit, a blood test is performed to determine your blood count to rule out anemia. If your levels are low, your health-care provider will advise you to take an iron supplement and to make sure that your diet is rich with green, leafy vegetables. Iron supplements tend to cause constipation, so drinking at least eight 8-ounce glasses of liquids each day, and increasing your fiber intake will help. Some women may need psyllium fiber supplements, such as Metamucil. Your blood levels are usually again monitored during the 24th to the 28th weeks of pregnancy, when you are also being tested for diabetes.

## Anesthesia

Use of local anesthetics to numb a specific area of the body is called regional, or local, anesthesia. Spinal, lumbar, caudal, and epidural anesthesia used for pain relief during labor and delivery are considered regional.

— *Epidural Anesthesia:* Epidural anesthesia is the most effective pain relief for labor and delivery. This type of anesthesia numbs you from the waist down, leaving you fully awake during your labor and delivery. An epidural is typically given after you are dilated to four centimeters. While you are seated or lying down, an anesthesiologist numbs the surface skin area, then inserts a tube between the vertebrae of your backbone. The tube is taped to your back to make it possible to give you a booster if you should need it, usually about every two hours. Your pain will typically disappear within 10 to 15 minutes (which feels like an eternity); on a rare occasion, the epidural is ineffective in relieving all of the pain. When you are ready to deliver, you may be given a "sitting dose." The tube is removed when the delivery is over. For a period of time following an epidural, you will be unable to walk or urinate; a catheter will be inserted into your bladder for continuous urinary drainage.

Epidural anesthesia is not without risks; epidurals have been associated with an arrest of labor and an increased incidence of forceps and vacuum deliveries. Complications of an epidural may include decreased blood pressure, which may cause a reduction in the fetus's heartbeat, and spinal headache.

— *Walking Epidural:* A walking epidural is a new, combined spinal-epidural block. With this procedure, a painkiller is injected into the spinal fluid instead of the administration of anesthesia. This type of block relieves pain, yet allows you to get up and walk around.

— *Spinal Anesthesia:* A spinal block completely numbs you and paralyzes you, leaving you unable to move for the duration of the effect of the anesthetic. It is given through a one-time injection into the cerebrospinal fluid surrounding your spinal column in your lower back. During pregnancy, the spinal block is reserved for C-sections, tubal sterilizations, and cervical cerclages. Complications of a spinal block may include hypotension and headaches. Rare complications include nerve injury and paralysis.

— _General Anesthesia:_ This produces a loss of consciousness and is typically reserved for emergency situations when there is no time to administer an epidural or spinal block.

Other less invasive types of anesthesia include: a paracervical block, where the anesthetic is directly injected into the cervix; a pudendal block, which numbs the vagina, rectum, and anus; and local infiltration, which is done before an episiotomy when the head of the baby is crowning, and only if you have received no other type of anesthesia during labor.

## Anxiety

During pregnancy when you feel anxious or nervous, try to relax, because it is believed that highly anxious women have a tendency toward restricted blood flow to the uterus. Use different relaxation techniques, such as meditation, breathing, yoga, and so on. Many studies have demonstrated the link between a mother's anxiety during pregnancy and low birth-weight babies.

## Apgar Scores

Newborns are given a numeric score at one minute and five minutes after birth. The score is tallied by careful observation of the heart rate, respiration, muscle tone, reflexes, and skin color, and ranges from 0 to 10. The higher the score, the better. Babies who experience distress during labor may have a low score at one minute but will improve after five minutes.

## Areola

The areola is the pigmented area surrounding the nipple. This area tends to widen and darken as your pregnancy progresses.

## Aromatherapy

Aromatherapy is the use of fragrance from essential oils, extracted from plants and herbs, to promote health. Essential oil fragrances can be very soothing and relaxing to the laboring mother. They may be added to water in a diffuser or used to massage the back and abdomen. Some recommended oils are neroli, lavender, and geranium. Aromatherapy has been successfully used to relieve stress, depression, and insomnia, among other ailments. *(Please note that certain aromatherapy oils are not suitable for pregnant women—consult with an aromatherapist before using any.)*

## Artificial Insemination

When a couple has failed at all attempts to conceive, they may turn to a health-care provider to try artificial insemination. In this method, the male partner's semen, or that of a donor, is injected into the cervix with a small syringe.

## Artificial Sweetener

Artificial sweeteners should be avoided during pregnancy.

## Aspirin

Aspirin should not be taken during pregnancy. Use of aspirin before conception and during pregnancy has been associated with babies who have lower-than-average IQs. It also increases bleeding.

## Augmentation of Labor

If labor is not progressing adequately due to poor-quality contractions, the drug pitocin may be given to enhance the strength of the contractions.

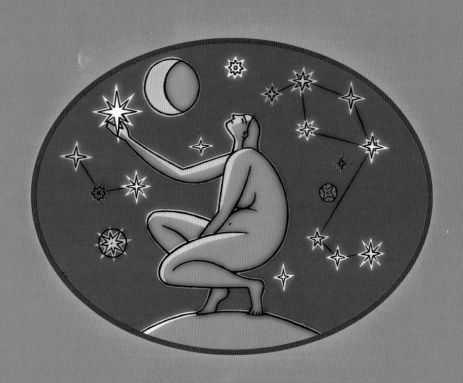

B

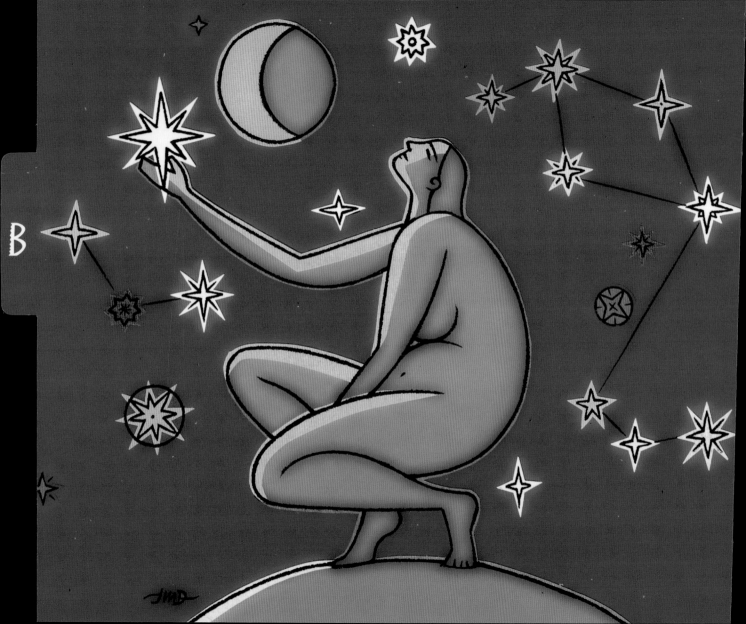

## Baby Shower

This is a joyous party given by your friends and family where you receive baby gifts. I am usually very practical when it comes to buying a gift for a baby shower. Even if I purchase something special for the baby, I always bring diapers and wipes because they are never too big or too small, and they are always appreciated.

## Backache

Backache is very common during pregnancy. It often consists of a dull pain in your middle or lower back, making it difficult to rise from a sitting or reclining position. During pregnancy, there is an excessive curvature of the spine and relaxed musculature causing lower back pain. Back pain may be the result of pregnancy changes as well as bad posture. Try to maintain good posture when walking, standing, exercising, and sitting. Avoid shoes with heels higher than one inch. If you must lift, bend from the knees while keeping your back straight.

During your first trimester, back pain associated with any vaginal bleeding or lower abdominal or pelvic cramping may be an indication of miscarriage or an ectopic pregnancy. During your second trimester, if back pain is accompanied by contractions, a feeling of pressure in your pelvic area, or an increase in vaginal discharge, this may be a sign of a late miscarriage due to cervical incompetency. Call your health-care provider immediately if this happens. If back pain occurs in your last trimester, this may be an indication that you are in labor. Back pain can be relieved by acupressure, acupuncture, biofeedback, chiropractic manipulations, and application of ice packs.

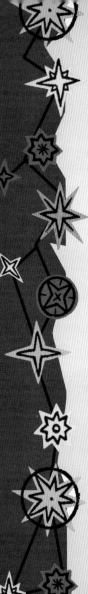

Backache, cont'd.

— _Lower Back Exercises:_

* **CAT STRETCH:** Get on your hands and knees, keeping your head in a straight line with your spine. Round your back up in a hump, like a cat, while tightening the muscles of your abdomen and buttocks. Allow your head to dip down, and slowly raise your head while relaxing your back. Return to the beginning position, and repeat these motions several times.

* **PELVIC TILT:** Stand straight with your back against a wall. Press your lower back into the wall by tightening your abdominal muscles.

## Bag of Water

Also called amniotic sac. Also see _Water Breaks._

## Biofeedback

During biofeedback, sensors are attached to your body, leading to a computer that registers electrical signals from your brain and muscles. These signals are translated into images and sound. Working with a therapist, you can learn how to affect these signals, and eventually learn how to control stress-related maladies such as anxiety, heart disease, hypertension, and urinary stress incontinence.

Biofeedback can be used during labor for pain relief, but it is not readily available and can be costly.

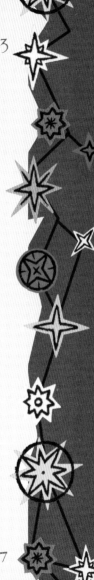

## Biophysical Profile

A biophysical profile is performed when more information is needed to confirm that the fetus is in good health. This profile includes a non-stress test and an ultrasound examination, where the amount of amniotic fluid, fetal movement, fetal muscle tone, and breathing movements are observed.

## Birth Attendants

Midwives, or "sage femmes," are the norm for routine deliveries in other countries. I was 11 years old when, in Haiti, I first assisted my mother in a home delivery. In the United States, a certified nurse-midwife or a family physician can be your birth attendant, but most deliveries are performed by obstetricians.

## Birth Defects

Birth defects increase with a mother's age. Women 35 years and older are at a higher risk for birth defects such as Down's syndrome, and should be offered genetic testing. Birth defects can also be associated with other factors, including:

* genetic transmission—accounting for about 20 to 25 percent of birth defects;

* chromosomal abnormalities—accounting for about 5 percent;

* drug exposure (illegal or prescribed medications), or radiation—2 to 3 percent;

* infection—about 2 percent; and

* possible combination of genetics and environmental factors account for the remaining birth defects.

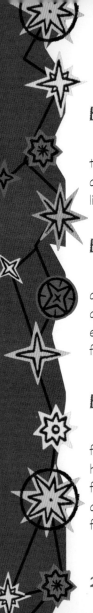

## Birthing Centers

Birthing centers offer a compromise between a hospital birth and a home birth. They offer a home-like setting, are located close to hospitals, and are typically run by midwives. The location is important because if complications arise, you'll want to be able to be transferred quickly for appropriate care. Only women who have very little risk of developing complications during pregnancy, labor, and delivery should use a birthing center.

## Birth Partner

Your birth partner may be the child's father or it may be a close friend or family member or a doula, but above all, it should be a caring, supportive, and reliable person. This is the individual who will attend childbirth classes with you and who will be there during your labor and delivery. The presence of a birth partner enhances a woman's sense of security during labor, helps her stick to her birth plan, and reduces the need for pain relief.

## Birth Plan

I advise you to document your wishes regarding medical intervention and indicate the birth plan you prefer. Put your questions and decisions about your labor and delivery in writing, and discuss them with your health-care provider. You'll need to be comfortable with, and have trust in, your provider, as it is important for this person to understand your desires and share your philosophy about your pregnancy. One word of caution: Since hospital deliveries are mostly performed by obstetricians in a large medical group, you may find yourself being delivered by a doctor you do not know, so having a written birth plan can be important.

# Bleeding

Bleeding may occur at any time during your pregnancy and is a sign that there may be a problem that should be evaluated by your health-care provider. Spotting may occur after intercourse.

During your first trimester, you may experience slight staining or bleeding around the time of your missed period, which is called implantation bleeding. Bleeding during your first trimester can be caused by cervical infection or abrasion, or it can be an early indication of a miscarriage or an ectopic pregnancy.

During your second trimester, any bleeding may be the sign of a late miscarriage due to cervical incompetency.

During your third trimester, bleeding may indicate placenta previa, where the afterbirth comes before the baby; or a placenta abruptio, where the placenta partially or completely covers the cervix.

Vaginal bleeding typically occurs for two to six weeks after childbirth; intercourse and tampon use should be avoided during this time. Sometimes there may be a transient period of bleeding, possibly heavy. If this bleeding does not subside within two hours, call your health-care provider to be evaluated for possible retention of placental tissue.

# Bleeding Gums

Due to the increased blood flow throughout your body, your gums may bleed easily during pregnancy. Brush your teeth with a soft toothbrush, and floss regularly to keep your gums healthy. You can also massage your gums periodically with your fingers. A natural remedy for bleeding includes chewing one teaspoon of papaya seeds three to four times a day, spitting them out after chewing them thoroughly.

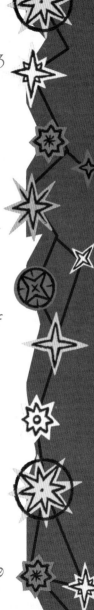

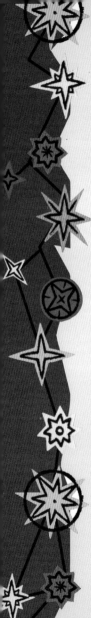

## Blurred Vision

Blurred vision is a symptom associated with pre-eclampsia. You should report this to your health-care provider immediately.

## Boy

The cute newborn baby with "outdoor plumbing."

## Bradley Methods

In these childbirth classes, couples learn about relaxation and breathing techniques. Doing what comes naturally is emphasized. This childbirth method is a combination of Lamaze and Dick-Read methods, with emphasis on the father as the primary labor coach.

## Braxton-Hicks Contractions

During the last weeks of pregnancy, your body is preparing itself for labor, and you may begin to feel cramps. Braxton-Hicks contractions occur during the last trimester of pregnancy and can last from 30 seconds to 2 minutes. These contractions are responsible for false labor.

As delivery approaches, these contractions become strong and increasingly regular.

## Breast

The female breast is an important element of a woman's sexuality, in addition to being the natural source of nutrition for a newborn. The breast consists of mammary glands, or milk glands, that are capable of producing milk. These glands empty into a system of ducts that lead to the nipple. These glands and ducts are surrounded by fatty tissue. The breast tissue extends into the armpit, where lymph nodes are present. Lymph nodes are bean-shaped structures that are scattered along the vessels of the lymph system. The nodes act as filters, collecting bacteria or cancer cells that may travel through the system. The size of a woman's breasts is determined by her genes (or her plastic surgeon).

By the time a woman has noticed a missed period, her breasts have become fuller and heavier, are sometimes sensitive to touch, are tender, and have increased in size due to the enlargement of the ducts and milk glands. The tenderness usually subsides as pregnancy progresses. The nipples and veins within the breast also become more prominent. Bra size often doubles during pregnancy, so it is important to wear a properly fitted bra that provides good support. The breasts can become hard, warm, and painful after childbirth. These symptoms can be relieved by cool compresses.

## Breast Cancer

Breast cancer can occur at any time, but could be missed during pregnancy because of the natural changes that occur. If you notice a lump during this time, do not disregard it as being due to the pregnancy. Have it checked by your health-care provider, and do not let anyone easily dismiss you. Each year, approximately 180,000 women are diagnosed with breast cancer. For about 4,000 of them, the diagnosis is made during pregnancy.

Having a history of breast cancer should not preclude a woman from becoming pregnant. According to a

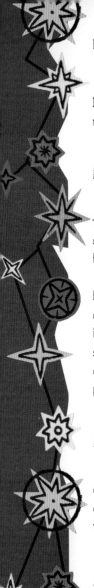

Breast Cancer, cont'd.

Danish study published in 1997, women who had a full-term pregnancy following breast cancer had a lower risk of death when compared with women who had no subsequent pregnancy.

## Breast-feeding

Breast milk is the best form of nutrition for the newborn; there is no substitute. I strongly recommend that every baby be breast-fed during the first six months. It's convenient—no bottle to warm up or wash—and above all, it's *free*. Children who have been breast-fed are less likely to suffer from infectious diseases, have less serious infections, fewer hospitalizations, and experience improved motor and mental development.

Also, an intense mother-infant bonding occurs during breast-feeding. Women who breast-feed their babies have a reduced risk of ovarian and premenopausal breast cancer, osteoporosis, and hip fractures, and lose less blood after childbirth. Fortunately, our society has become more open to women breast-feeding in public. Immediately after, or within a few hours of birth, your baby will be placed on your breast to learn to suck. Suckling is necessary in order to initiate your milk production. Consider enrolling in a breast-feeding class before your baby is born. While breast-feeding, you should continue with your prenatal vitamins, drink plenty of fluids, and eat a calcium-rich diet. You may wish to consider calcium supplements.

## Breast Implants

Some women elect a surgical procedure using implants to augment breast size. These implants consist of a silicone bag, filled with either saline or silicone gel. To insert the implants, an incision is made in the crease under the breast, under the arm, or around the nipple. Implants are positioned either under or over the chest muscle. You should still be able to breast-feed if you have breast implants.

## Breast Lump

Many women have a condition sometimes erroneously referred to as fibrocystic disease, a condition marked by lumpy, painful, and cystic breasts. This is the most common condition associated with benign breast lumps. A great number of women experience fibrocystic changes, or breasts that feel lumpy. These women may notice swelling, tenderness, or even some pain before, and sometimes during, their menstrual cycle. These symptoms can worsen with pregnancy.

## Breast Pump

If unable to breast-feed on schedule, a breast pump may be used to express milk to be stored for a later feeding.

## Breathing Techniques

The goal of these natural techniques is to relax the mind and the body during pregnancy, labor, and delivery. Breathing exercises can be effective for relieving pain and anxiety during labor and delivery. Take slow deep breaths, inhale deeply (filling the entire diaphragm), and hold for a few seconds. Then release the air very gradually through your mouth.

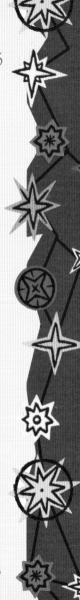

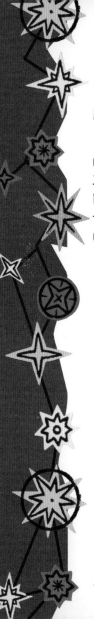

## Breech Delivery

A breech delivery is a condition where the baby is positioned feet or buttocks first, instead of head first (vertex). This occurs in 3 to 7 percent of pregnancies. The fetus is usually settled into the pelvis by the 37th week of pregnancy. Twelve percent of these babies do convert spontaneously from breech to vertex. Relaxation techniques can be used to relax the lower abdomen and lower uterine segment, allowing the baby to turn. A breech baby may also be turned around by a procedure known as external cephalic version (ECV). Most breech babies are delivered by cesarean section.

## Caffeine

Caffeine is a stimulant that can enter the growing fetus's bloodstream. Most studies have not determined that caffeine harms the pregnant woman, but a few studies have found a relationship between caffeine and an increased risk of miscarriage and decreased fertility. Since the "safe" amount of caffeine during pregnancy is not known, drink no more than the equivalent of two to three cups of coffee daily.

Caffeine is also present in chocolate, cola drinks, tea, and some over-the-counter medications.

## Calcium

Calcium is a mineral necessary for the healthy development of strong bones. A pregnant and lactating woman should consume 1,200 to 1,500 mg of calcium per day. Your diet should be your first choice for increasing calcium intake. You can do so by eating more leafy green vegetables and legumes and calcium-fortified products. You may fortify other food by adding a tablespoon or two of nonfat dry milk to baked goods, hot beverages, or casseroles. Dairy products such as milk, yogurt, and cheese are good sources of calcium. Stick to a low-fat version of these products. Broccoli, turnip greens, and canned salmon with bones are great sources of calcium as well.

If you cannot get the recommended amount of calcium through your diet, you may take a calcium supplement; choose supplements containing calcium citrate, asporotate, or carbonate. Calcium absorption is enhanced when it is taken in smaller doses, twice each day, versus one large dose.

## Carpal Tunnel Syndrome (CTS)

This condition is also a common side effect of pregnancy, due to swelling. Symptoms include numbness, tingling, and pain in the palm, thumb, index finger, middle finger, and half of the ring finger. The pinkie is not affected. To relieve CTS, get a carpal tunnel splint at your drug store, and put it on before going to bed.

## Car Seat

You will need to purchase an infant car seat made to fit newborns in order to bring your baby home from the hospital. It's the law!

## Centimeters

The unit of measurement used to describe cervical dilation (opening).

## Certified Nurse-Midwife (CNM)

This person is a nurse with additional state-certified training in midwifery. Midwives can attend home and hospital deliveries. During deliveries that are attended by midwives, laboring women typically require less pain medication, receive fewer episiotomies, and are less likely to deliver by cesarean section.

As an intern in Jamaica, I received training from nurse-midwives in a technique to deliver babies of all sizes without an episiotomy. The basis of the technique is patience and cooperation between mother and midwife. What a difference I saw when I arrived in the United States for my postgraduate training in obstetrics and gynecology!

## Cervical Cerclage

This term refers to a procedure in which a mesh or suture is placed underneath the superficial layer of the cervix, at the level of the junction with the uterus, and tied to keep the cervix closed. The suture is removed around the 38th week of pregnancy, if labor progresses, or if there is an indication of an infection.

## Cervical Dilation

During labor, the cervix begins to thin and open (dilate), progressing to fully dilated at about ten centimeters. This dilation allows the baby to pass through the vagina. Typically, you will be checked periodically to evaluate your dilation progress, and findings will be recorded on your chart.

## Cervical Effacement

Before the cervix is able to dilate, it needs to thin out, or efface. The degree of effacement is expressed as a percentage. Example: The cervix is 50 percent effaced, or fully effaced.

## Cervical Incompetency

In this condition, the cervix is too weak to hold the increasing weight of the growing fetus, and it dilates prematurely and painlessly, usually after the 14th week of pregnancy. The cause is unknown but has been correlated to women born with insufficient connective tissue to hold their cervixes closed. Abnormal cervixes occur among women whose mothers took a medication known as diethylstilbestrol (DES) during their

39

pregnancies. (This drug was prescribed to prevent morning sickness and miscarriage.) Incompetency is also associated with some cervical surgeries, such as conization for precancerous lesions of the cervix or cervical cancer. This condition is difficult to diagnose during first pregnancies. Among women with cervical incompetency, pregnancy loss can be prevented by inserting a cervical cerclage after the 13th week of pregnancy.

## Cervical Ripening

When labor must be induced and the cervix is unfavorable due to being long, thick, and closed, medication may need to be applied to the cervix to soften it.

## Cervix

The cervix is the lowermost portion of the uterus, a narrow neckline that opens into the vagina. This opening dilates during childbirth and is the site from which a Pap smear is taken. After fertilization, the number of mucous glands and blood vessels increases, making the cervix soft and spongy and giving it a violet hue. During pregnancy, the mucous glands also create a mucous plug that seals the cervical opening.

## Cesarean Section

Sometimes it is necessary to deliver a baby through the mother's abdomen instead of via the vagina. The United States has one of the highest rates of cesarean sections, or C-sections. The increase in the rate of C-sections is mostly due to the overuse of technology and the medicalization of childbirth fueled by the fear of lawsuits if a baby is not perfect. In the United States, one in four babies is delivered by

C-section; the incidence is higher among the most educated. C-sections are sometimes scheduled in advance.

A C-section is a major surgery associated with bleeding, infection, longer recovery in the hospital and at home, and less maternal involvement with the delivery. During a C-section, your pubic hair will be shaved, and a Foley catheter will be inserted into your bladder for continuous urinary drainage. Scheduled C-sections are generally performed with a spinal block. General anesthesia, where the mother is unconscious, is reserved for emergency cases.

## Childbirth Classes

Attending childbirth classes with the baby's father, a doula, or a close friend as a birth partner, is recommended. These classes will help you mentally prepare for labor and delivery. This is also a way to involve the father more and help him feel better about the pregnancy. Together, you can learn about labor, childbirth, breathing and relaxation techniques, and muscle control in order to cope with the pain and stress of childbirth. Such classes include Lamaze, Bradley, and the Grantly Dick-Read method.

## Chiropractic Medicine

Chiropractic care has been well documented as an effective method for pain relief (back pain, headaches, and sciatica), as well as a means of increasing spinal flexibility and integrity. Chiropractic manipulation has been very helpful to my pregnant patients suffering from back pain.

## Chlamydia

Chlamydia is a sexually transmitted disease caused by a bacteria that is transmitted by an infected person during sexual intercourse. Men may experience a painful discharge from the penis, burning upon urination, and sometimes burning and itching at the tip of the penis. Unfortunately, up to 20 percent of males with the disease show no symptoms. Chlamydia can be treated with oral antibiotics. A woman may have a whitish or yellowish vaginal discharge that may be heavy. Up to 75 percent of women with chlamydia have no symptoms. Without treatment, chlamydia can result in pelvic inflammatory disease and infertility. Children born to infected women can have eye infections and pneumonia.

## Chloasma

Also known as the "mask of pregnancy," chloasma appears during pregnancy as brownish patches covering the nose, cheeks, and forehead. This rash usually disappears after delivery.

## Choosing a Name

Remember that children with common names tend to be better accepted by, and more popular among, their peers.

## Chorionic Villus Sampling (CVS)

A sample of cells is taken from placental tissue under ultrasound guidance to analyze the genetic material of fetal cells. It is usually performed between the 9th and 12th week of pregnancy when there is a need to rule out a chromosomal defect.

## Chromosomes

Chromosomes are threadlike structures in a living cell that contain the cell's genetic information. Normally there are 46 chromosomes in a cell.

## Circumcision

Circumcision is the removal of a piece of tissue called the foreskin, or prepuce, that covers the tip (glans) of the penis. There is no medical indication to do a circumcision at birth—this is a cultural and religious decision. It is usually performed during the first 48 hours after birth, and in the Jewish tradition, a special ceremony called the "bris" is held the eighth day after birth of a boy. There is a strong advocacy to use local anesthesia to avoid undue pain to the infant during the surgery of circumcision. Good personal hygiene offers all the advantages of circumcision, without surgery.

## Colds

Colds and flu-like symptoms can and do occur during pregnancy. Check with your health-care provider prior to taking any over-the-counter medication. Natural home remedies include:

* inhaling steam from a kettle of boiling water that contains a drop or two of menthol, or peppermint oil;

* using clove, cinnamon, or lavender oils in steam to relieve bronchial congestion;

Colds, cont'd.

* drinking hot beverages and gargling with warm salt water to treat a sore throat;
* getting plenty of rest and keeping your body hydrated by drinking eight glasses of fluid each day; and . . .

. . . don't forget the tried-and-true remedy: warm chicken soup!

## Colostrum

This is a highly nutritious, yellowish liquid that the newborn infant suckles on until your breast milk comes in. Some women may experience a slight discharge of colostrum as early as the first trimester of pregnancy. For the first three to four days, the newborn will feed on colostrum. Colostrum is low in fat and carbohydrates, and high in protein and antibodies, which are protective substances that fight infection.

## Conception

The union of an egg and a sperm.

## Congenital

A condition or disease that is present at birth.

## Constipation

During pregnancy, digestion is twice as sluggish as normal, often resulting in constipation. Constipation is the passage of hard and infrequent stools. Many pregnant women, especially those who take iron supplements, may suffer from constipation. Drink at least eight 8-ounce glasses of liquids each day, and consume a high-fiber diet including dried fruits and bran. Some women may need psyllium fiber supplements such as Metamucil. Regular exercise also helps relieve constipation. Laxatives should be avoided.

## Contractions

During labor, the muscles of your uterus contract in a regular fashion, causing cervical thinning and opening, which helps to push your baby out of the vagina. When a woman is in active labor, contractions occur two to three minutes apart and last about a minute. To time your contractions, write down the number of minutes that pass from the beginning of one contraction to the beginning of the next. You are in labor if your contractions are at least three to five minutes apart for at least one hour, and they appear to be getting stronger.

## Corpus Luteum

A yellow glandular mass formed by an ovarian follicle after ovulation. The corpus luteum nourishes the embryo during the first 12 weeks of pregnancy until the placenta is ready to take over.

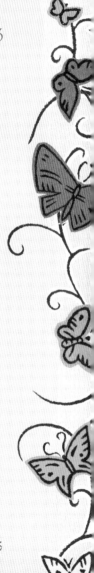

45

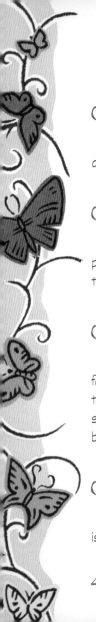

## Cough

For a cough due to a cold, a steamy shower, a bath with eucalyptus oil, or a glass of warm water with or without a teaspoon of vinegar may provide relief.

## Cramps

Cramps are common a few days after childbirth ("afterpains"), as the uterus contracts to its pre-pregnancy size. Cramps are stronger among women who breast-feed and may be relieved by analgesics that will not affect the newborn baby. Contractions may be perceived as cramps.

## Cravings

Cravings are a common symptom of pregnancy. When they are strong enough, you will send the future father out into the wee hours of the night, searching for strange combinations of food. Cravings may be due to a need for a particular nutrient or mineral. In my native Haitian culture, there is a belief that if you crave something while pregnant, you should avoid touching your body until the sensation is gone; otherwise, the baby will be born with a birthmark wherever you first touch yourself.

## Crowning

During birth when half of the baby's head is outside of the vagina, the baby is said to be crowning. This is also the time when the episiotomy is performed.

# Cystitis

Infections of the urinary tract (which encompasses the bladder and kidneys) are common during pregnancy. An infection of the bladder, or cystitis, is more common and is characterized by a burning sensation, pain while urinating, frequent urination, and sometimes blood in the urine. If cystitis is not properly treated, it can result in a kidney infection.

# Cytomegalovirus (CMV)

About 60 to 70 percent of the population is infected with this virus but is unaware of it. This virus is spread through sexual intercourse and through the saliva. It rarely causes serious problems in an adult; however, if a woman becomes infected during pregnancy, she can transmit CMV to her fetus, possibly causing birth defects, blindness, and even death, in a small percentage of cases.

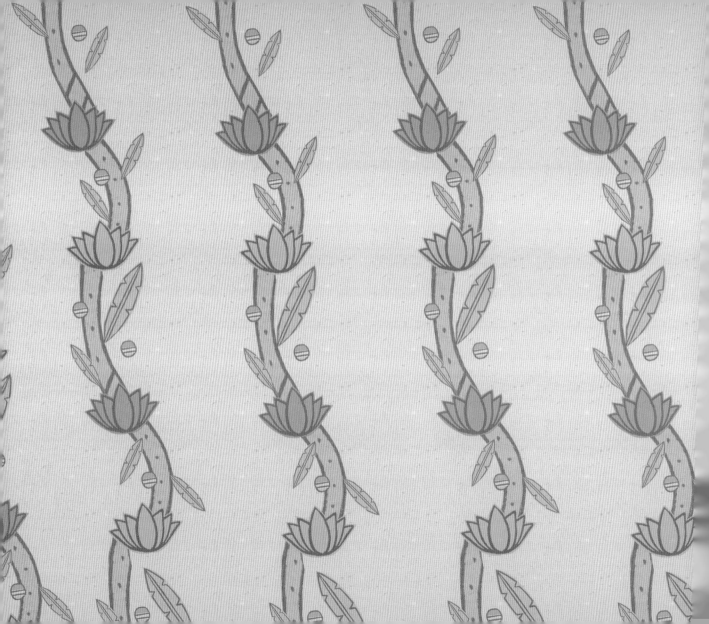

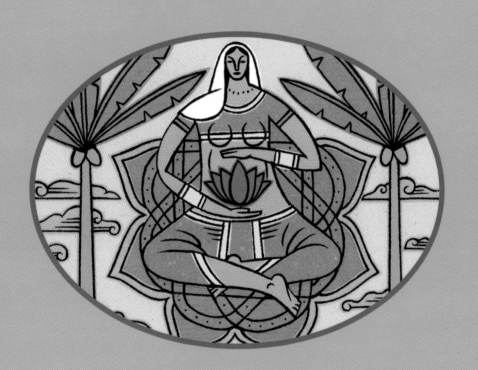

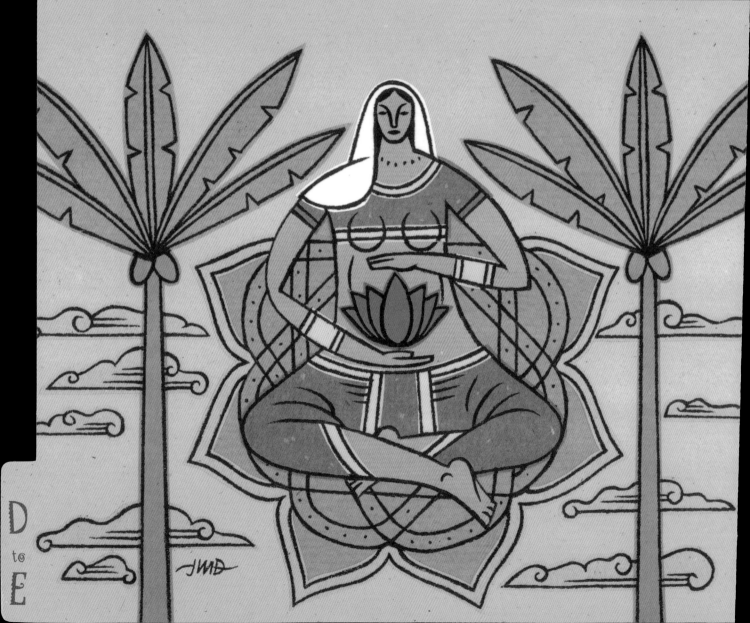

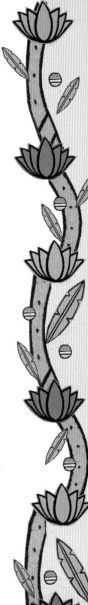

## Danger Signals

If any of the following symptoms occur, contact your health-care provider immediately:

- Excessive vomiting.
- Vaginal bleeding. During the early stages of pregnancy, this could indicate a miscarriage or an ectopic pregnancy; later in the pregnancy, this could indicate the abnormal separation of the placenta.
- Excessive weight gain in a short period of time; or excessive swelling of the hands, feet, or face.
- Contractions close together when it's not yet time to give birth.
- Fluid from the vagina.
- Constant headaches.
- Blurred vision.
- Fever and chills.
- If you sense that the baby is not as active as it should be.

## Dating of the Pregnancy

How far along you are in your pregnancy is calculated in terms of weeks, not months, since all tests are performed according to how many weeks along you are in the pregnancy. To discover exactly how far along you are at any point in time, ask your health-care provider to tell you when you complete a week of pregnancy. For instance, let's say your tenth week of pregnancy ends on a Wednesday. Each subsequent Wednesday will add one more week to your gestation—that is, you will be 11 weeks on the following

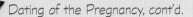

Wednesday. In the meantime, you can say that you are ten-plus weeks.

If you know exactly how far along you are, this is information that can be important to know when you arrive at the hospital, call your doctor's office, or when you are out of town and your medical records are not readily available. This information can also help your medical provider differentiate between an emergency and a non-emergency situation. If you are having regular contractions at 38 weeks, you will be instructed to go to the hospital when the contractions become frequent; however, if you are only 35 weeks, you are in premature labor and need to be evaluated right away.

# Delivery

The baby finally arrives after months of expectation (which can seem like an eternity)! Once the head is out, the nose and the mouth are suctioned to remove any mucus that could block the baby's airway. A small tube attached to a suction pump may be used to get the baby ready for its first breath if there is any indication of meconium, a greenish-tinged amniotic fluid that suggests that the fetus may have defecated in utero. After the delivery of the head, the shoulders and the rest of the body follow. The long-awaited moment has arrived: "It's a boy," or "It's a girl." At this point, it won't much matter what the sex is—you are just happy that it's over. The newborn may be placed on your abdomen, and the cord will then be clamped. If you have chosen the Leboyer method, your birth attendant will wait until the cord has stopped pulsating before clamping it. The cord will then be cut by the baby's father, by your birth attendant, or by whomever you choose.

Your new baby may look funny with its little pointed head; its body covered with waxy, white particles called vernix; or mixed with blood if you had an episiotomy. If meconium was present, your baby may actually have a greenish hue.

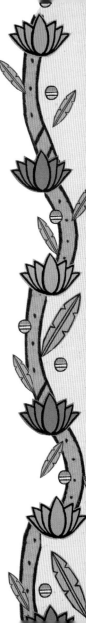

In the case of fetal distress, a pediatrician, neonatologist, or nurse will place your baby in a warmer next to the delivery bed. The delivery team will continue to clean, suction, and stimulate your baby. Your baby will also be observed for the Apgar scores.

Cord blood will be obtained to check for the baby's blood type. Some blood may be saved for future medical use. The placenta, or afterbirth, will be delivered. Your health-care provider may have to manually remove the placenta. Your uterus may then be manually explored to make sure that there are no pieces remaining. If you had an episiotomy, it will then be repaired.

## Delivery Room

Long ago, women labored in a labor room, then were wheeled into a delivery room. After delivery, the woman was transported to a recovery room and then to her final postpartum room where she stayed until discharge. Today, most hospitals have fancy labor-delivery-recovery and postpartum (LDRP) rooms where you are admitted, go into labor, deliver, recover, and stay until you are able to go home with your new baby.

## Dental Care

During your pregnancy, continue with regular dental hygiene, including brushing and flossing. You may notice bleeding gums, which is caused by the increased blood flow. Use a soft toothbrush to minimize bleeding. Keep your scheduled cleaning appointments. In the event of an emergency, your dentist can consult with your health-care provider regarding your treatment plan. Dental x-rays are allowed as long as you are covered with a lead apron.

# Depression

Women who suffer from depression should be treated during their pregnancy as well as during the postpartum period. There is no evidence that drugs such as the selective serotonin reuptake inhibitors (SSRIs) have any adverse effects on the infant. To the contrary, fetuses exposed to untreated maternal depression in utero may be at increased risk of premature birth and low birth weight.

Maternal depression also has an adverse impact on infant attachment and infant development.

# Diabetes

This is a disease caused by failure of the body to produce insulin or use insulin efficiently, resulting in high levels of sugar in the bloodstream and urine. During pregnancy, some women may be prone to develop gestational diabetes, where the hormones produced by the placenta alter the usual manner in which insulin is produced and utilized. Gestational diabetes can be detected by a glucose screen, usually performed around the 24th to 28th week of gestation. If you are overweight, are over 35, have delivered a large baby in the past, or have a family history of diabetes, your health-care provider may decide to test you earlier. Gestational diabetes usually disappears after delivery. Diabetic women who are pregnant require close medical supervision.

# Dieting

Some women may be unhappy about their weight gain during pregnancy. Dieting is not recommended during pregnancy, since losing weight at that time could harm your unborn child. Women who breast-feed their newborn baby lose their pregnancy weight faster than those who do not.

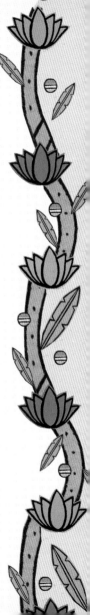

## Dilation and Curettage (D&C)

This is a medical procedure to scrape away part of the uterine lining (endometrium), to remove abnormal cells, remove the product of a miscarriage, or perform an abortion.

## Dizziness

Also described as a "spinning sensation," dizziness results from the increased blood supply to the uterus, which deprives the brain of blood. During pregnancy, there may also be a reduction in a woman's blood pressure. If you stand or move too quickly—or stand up for too long—you may feel dizzy, so don't do it.

## Doppler

This is a hand-held soundwave stethoscope that enables your health-care provider to hear the fetal heartbeat after the tenth week of gestation.

## Douching

Douching is not necessary for a woman to keep her vagina clean, whether or not she is pregnant. Douching should be avoided during pregnancy because it can cause a fatal air embolism.

## Doula

A doula is a female support person, specially trained to provide emotional support to the laboring mother. This support makes things easier for the mother and her partner, shortens labor, and decreases the chance of a cesarean section and the need for pain medication and epidural anesthesia. Women who receive a doula's support feel more accepting of their infant and more capable of caring for him or her.

## Down's Syndrome

This is a very common chromosomal abnormality in which the baby has 47 instead of the normal 46 chromosomes. It can occur in one out of every 600 to 800 births. This is a genetic abnormality that results in medical problems such as heart defects, mental retardation, and abnormal facial features. The risk of Down's syndrome increases from 1.9 percent per 1,000 pregnancies at age 20, to 5.2 percent per 1,000 pregnancies at age 35, and 47.6 percent per 1,000 pregnancies in a 45-year-old woman.

## Drugs (recreational)

The use of illegal or street drugs is unhealthy whether or not you are pregnant. Recreational drug use should be stopped for six months to a year before you decide to conceive. Cocaine use may decrease the concentration of sperm in the semen and prevent pregnancy. Marijuana, a drug that has been touted as being harmless, injects more tar and nicotine into the smoker's lungs than regular cigarette smoking does. Marijuana may also change the embryo's genetic makeup, thus causing birth defects.

During pregnancy, the majority of drugs that are used by the mother reach the baby by way of the placenta, the organ responsible for the baby's nutrition. When a pregnant woman abuses drugs such as cocaine and crystal methamphetamine, she is at risk for premature labor. The infant is at risk of being addicted at birth and may suffer from brain, heart, kidney, and intestinal problems. Drug use may also increase the risk that the baby will have a stroke or be stillborn.

## Due Date

When an accurate estimated date of delivery or "due date" is known, problems such as preterm and postterm labor, and lack of fetal growth, can easily be evaluated. Knowledge of the due date is also important for the application and interpretation of certain tests performed during the prenatal period. An accurate due date is the most important factor in helping your health-care provider diagnose an overdue baby.

A regular pregnancy term is about 40 weeks (or ten lunar months). An unborn baby is mature and ready to be born at plus or minus two weeks of the due date. An ultrasound scan may be ordered during your pregnancy to confirm your due date. Your due date may change after an ultrasound is done. Most fetuses grow at the same rate until mid-pregnancy, then factors such as gender, genetics, phenotype, and environment affect how big or small the fetus will become.

## Dystocia

This is a general term used to describe the failure of labor to progress to a normal vaginal delivery.

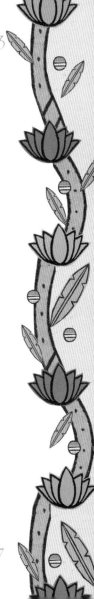

## Eclampsia

When a woman diagnosed with pre-eclampsia begins to develop seizures, she has developed eclampsia. Eclampsia is characterized by convulsions, cerebral hemorrhage, and coma, and it can be fatal to both mother and fetus.

## Ectopic Pregnancy

In this particular situation, the fertilized egg attaches to, and begins to grow outside of, the uterus or womb. In most cases, it occurs in one of the Fallopian tubes. Signs of an ectopic pregnancy may include: cramping or sharp, one-sided pelvic pain (so painful that one may faint); shoulder pain; spotting; or bleeding. These symptoms usually occur before the eighth week of pregnancy. An unsuspected ectopic pregnancy may lead to hemorrhage, shock, and if untreated, to collapse and death. Ectopic pregnancy is one of the leading causes of maternal death in the United States.

## Edema

Edema refers to the fluid retention that is common during late pregnancy, but it can also be an indication of trouble. If you notice excessive weight gain over a short period of time, or excessive swelling of your hands, feet, or face, call your health-care provider immediately.

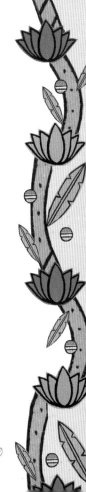

# Effacement

Thinning out of the cervix.

# Egg

Pregnancy begins with conception, when a sperm penetrates a mature egg (ovum), in a process called fertilization. An egg has an average life span of 24 hours. If the egg is not fertilized during this time period, it dissolves within the body.

# Electronic Fetal Monitoring (EFM)

This equipment is used to monitor your contractions, and the heartbeat of the fetus, during labor.

# Embryo

The fetus is referred to as an embryo during the first eight weeks of your pregnancy.

# Endometrium

The endometrium is the inner lining of the uterus, which builds up and is shed each month as a normal part of your menstrual cycle.

# Epidural

Epidural anesthesia is the most effective pain relief for labor and delivery. This type of anesthesia numbs you from the waist down, leaving you fully awake during your labor and delivery. An epidural is typically given after you are dilated to four centimeters. While you are seated or lying down, an anesthesiologist numbs the surface skin area, then inserts a tube between the vertebrae of your backbone. The tube is taped to your back to make it possible to give you a booster if you should need it, usually every two hours. Your pain will typically disappear within 10 to 15 minutes (which feels like an eternity); on a rare occasion, the epidural is ineffective at relieving all of the pain. When you are ready to deliver, you may be given a "sitting dose." The tube is removed when the delivery is over. For a period of time following an epidural, you will be unable to walk or urinate; a catheter will be inserted into your bladder for continuous urinary drainage.

Epidural anesthesia is not without risks; epidurals have been associated with an arrest of labor and an increased incidence of forceps and vacuum deliveries. Complications of an epidural may include decreased blood pressure, which may cause a reduction in the fetus's heartbeat, and spinal headache.

— _Walking Epidural:_ A walking epidural is a new, combined spinal-epidural block. With this procedure, a painkiller is injected into the spinal fluid, instead of the administration of anesthesia. This type of block relieves pain, yet allows you to get up and walk around.

# Episiotomy

An episiotomy is a surgical cut into the perineum to facilitate the delivery of your baby. Episiotomies are performed in more than 60 percent of all vaginal deliveries; however, there is no data to support routine episiotomy. The use of episiotomy is controversial. Some health-care providers, including myself, believe that an episiotomy should only be performed when necessary. Given enough time, the perineum naturally

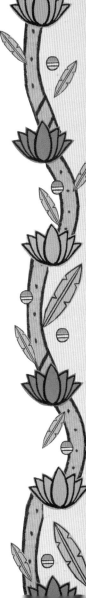

stretches. An episiotomy is necessary in the case of fetal distress, or when the baby's head is too large and may cause severe tears. A local anesthetic is used to numb the perineum when the baby is crowning only if you have not received another form of anesthesia during labor.

If you have had an episiotomy, you can promote the healing process by placing a cloth-covered ice pack over the perineum during the first 24 hours. After that period, a hot water bottle, or 20-minute sitz baths, will help speed the healing process. Episiotomy stitches can take up to two weeks to heal and dissolve.

## Estimated Date of Confinement (EDC)

The estimated date of confinement is the expected time of delivery at term. This date usually falls between 38 to 42 weeks after your last menstrual period (LMP). Your EDC may also be calculated from ultrasound findings.

## Exercise

You should not have to interrupt your current exercise routine during your pregnancy, except if you feel tired or if your health-care provider has recommended strict bed rest. It is perfectly safe for you to begin an exercise program during pregnancy (even if you haven't been exercising regularly up to that point), provided that the exercise is moderate, your pregnancy is normal, and you heed your body's pregnancy-related limits. It is important to remember that, when pregnant, part of your oxygen intake is being diverted to your baby. While moderate aerobic exercise is fine, contact sports and exhaustive aerobic exercise should be avoided, as they increase your need for oxygen at the expense of your unborn child. *Remember to stop exercising when you become tired.*

A pregnant woman should not exercise if she experiences any of the following:

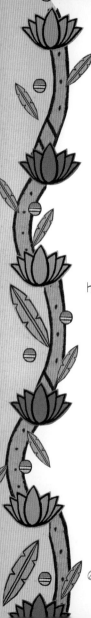

Exercise, cont'd.

* High blood pressure related to pregnancy.

* Premature rupture of the bag of water.

* Premature labor during a prior or current pregnancy.

* A cervical cerclage: a weak cervix that has been surgically tied due to premature labor or prior miscarriage.

* Persistent bleeding during the second or third trimester.

* Signs of lack of growth of the fetus.

Women who exercise in the postpartum months retain less weight, feel better about themselves, and have less difficulty adapting to the demands of being a new mother.

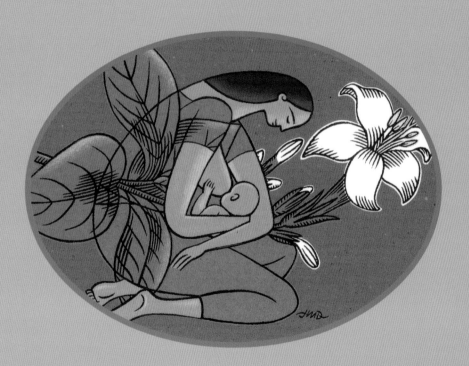

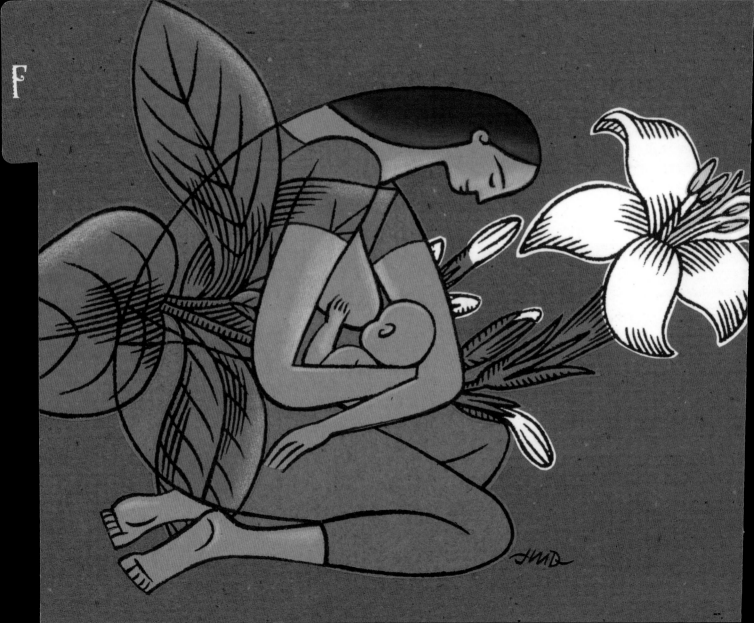

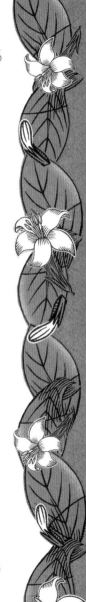

## Failure to Progress

When labor stalls and the cervix stops dilating, pitocin, a drug used to stimulate contractions, may be given intravenously. In some cases, a cesarean section may be necessary.

## Fallopian Tube

The Fallopian tubes protrude like a pair of arms from the top of your uterus. It is through these tubes that the egg travels on its way from the ovary to the uterus, where fertilization may occur. Each tube is fairly mobile and measures approximately four inches long.

## False Labor

Uterine contractions, in the absence of a cervical change, are called false labor. Do not be disappointed, as labor will eventually happen. My grandmother used to say, "Everything shall come to an end." During false labor, contractions are:

* irregular and do not get closer together;
* weak and do not get stronger;
* stopped when there is a change of position or movement; and
* felt in the abdomen.

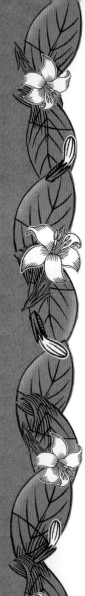

## Family Physician

A family physician is a doctor with training in all aspects of internal medicine and primary care, including obstetrics and pediatrics. Some family physicians follow pregnant women during their labor and delivery; however, if there are complications, or if a cesarean section is required, an obstetrician will be summoned.

## Family Planning

You'll need to think about family planning while you are pregnant. It is usually advised that you wait approximately 18 months to two years before you try to become pregnant again. If you do not want to have more children, you may want to consider permanent sterilization.

## Father

Also called Dad, or the sperm donor. Pregnancy is nature's way of testing the strength and love of one prospective parent for the other. With all the hormonal changes, a woman's emotions are on a roller coaster, so the father should be patient and know when to stay quiet. Dad, be a willing participant in childbirth exercises. During labor, agree with her "always." Just be supportive and caring throughout the entire process.

After childbirth, help her feel better about herself, congratulate her for small improvements, and tell her that she is doing a great job. Be willing to help with the baby's care. Don't feel rejected if she is not interested in sex, even after her six-week checkup. Try not to become jealous if, at first, the baby reacts to its mother more than it does to you.

## Fatigue

Fatigue is one of the most commonly reported symptoms, especially early in the pregnancy, due to the hard work occurring within your body. Fatigue is most common during the first and third trimesters. Try to be well rested.

## Feet

Puffiness of the feet is common during pregnancy. If your feet are swollen, avoid standing for long periods of time. Extreme cases may be associated with pre-eclampsia. Massage and reflexology can be utilized to increase circulation. Also, try to avoid salty food.

## Fertile Days

There are specific days in the middle of your menstrual cycle when you are most likely to conceive; these are called your fertile days. Here's how to calculate the most fertile period during your cycle. Let's assume that you are like the average woman and have a 28-day cycle. Ovulation usually occurs about 14 days before your next period, or day 14. Subtract three days from that day of ovulation (14 - 3 = 11). Also add three days (14 + 3 = 17). Your most fertile time is, therefore, from day 11 through day 17 of your cycle. (Day 1 is the first day of bleeding.) If you are trying to become pregnant, engage in sexual intercourse without contraception during these days; every other day is often enough. There is no need to make a marathon of it—unless that is desired! Eggs live for an average of 24 hours, and sperm live about 48 hours, with some especially tenacious sperm living longer than 72 hours. Most important, try not to worry, let Mother Nature take its course, and have fun!

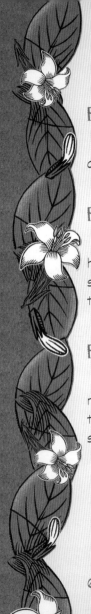

# Fertility

A woman's fertility, or capability of getting pregnant, reaches its peak at about 24 years of age, and continues to decline until she enters menopause at around age 50.

# Fertility Drugs

Fertility drugs are used to help infertile women ovulate. Typically, when a woman ovulates on her own, her ovaries release only one mature egg at a time. Fertility drugs prompt many eggs to mature at the same time. These drugs are generally used during natural intercourse that is timed to coincide with ovulation, intrauterine insemination, or in-vitro fertilization.

# Fertilization

Fertilization occurs when the tenacious sperm penetrates the mature egg. After fertilization, the inner membranes of the ovum are altered by enzymes, making it impossible for more sperm to enter. The nuclei of the egg and sperm each contain 23 chromosomes. Their union results in one fertilized egg with 46 chromosomes, essential for a healthy offspring.

# Fetal Alcohol Syndrome

When a pregnant woman abuses alcohol, she increases her risk of having a spontaneous abortion. Alternately, she may cause irreparable damage to her growing fetus in the form of fetal alcohol syndrome, which can include mental retardation and physical abnormalities. You should avoid alcohol while you are trying to conceive and during your pregnancy. While breast-feeding, you should keep your intake moderate.

# Fetal Capillary Blood Sampling

Your health-care provider may wish to obtain a sample of blood from the fetus while you are in labor in the event of fetal distress.

# Fetal Distress

Continuous fetal heart-rate monitoring may reveal specific signs that the fetus is in distress. This is typically a sign that the fetus isn't getting enough oxygen, and if it should persist, a cesarean section will probably be performed.

# Fetal Fibronectin

If you are admitted to the hospital with clinical symptoms of premature labor, you will be confined to bed rest, and you will receive vigorous drug treatments. Some women will experience the clinical symptoms of premature labor but do not progress to preterm delivery. For these women, a test for fetal fibronectin may be performed to differentiate women who are truly in premature labor.

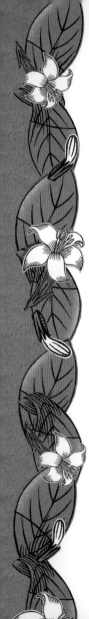

## Fetal Heart Rate Monitoring

Fetal heart rate monitoring can be performed with a stethoscope or by electronic methods during your labor.

## Fetal Heart Tone (FHT)

This is the fetus's heartbeat as heard with an instrument through your abdominal wall. The fetus's heart rate varies between 120 and 160 beats per minute.

## Fetal Position

Fetal position refers to the relationship of the fetus to the mother. Among 97 percent of pregnancies, the head is correctly positioned downward (cephalic presentation, or vertex).

## Fetal Station

Fetal station is a measure of the degree of descent of the presenting part of the fetus through the birth canal.

## Fetoscopy

Viewing a fetus with a fiberoptic lens in order to detect abnormalities is called fetoscopy. This procedure is performed only on rare occasions, and usually after the 15th week.

## Fetus

After your 12th week of pregnancy, until delivery, the baby is referred to as a fetus.

## Fever

High body temperatures, greater than 102 degrees Fahrenheit, should be avoided during your pregnancy, and especially during your first trimester, when excessively high temperatures in the developing embryo may be associated with damage to the nervous system. Accordingly, spas, saunas, Jacuzzis, whirlpools, hot tubs, and hot baths, where temperatures can be extremely high, should be avoided. Lukewarm baths, however, are soothing and relaxing.

## Fibroids

Fibroids are benign uterine tumors that may interfere with conception and implantation and may cause an abnormal fetal presentation, dystocia, placenta previa, placenta accreta, and postpartum hemorrhage.

## Flatulence

Flatulence, or excess gas, is extremely common during pregnancy because the intestines tend to be more sluggish. Avoid gassy foods such as beans, cabbage, onions, and fried foods.  Peppermints and soothing hot drinks can be helpful. Avoid chewing gum and drinking with straws in order to reduce the intake of air through the mouth.

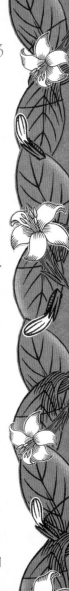

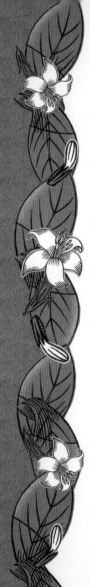

## Fluid Retention

Fluid retention occurs due to increased blood volume during pregnancy. You may notice the effects of fluid retention in your face, fingers, ankles, and feet. It may worsen in warm weather. Fluid retention may also be caused by the failure of your body to eliminate fluids due to cardiac, renal, or metabolic disease; or high levels of salt in your body. To prevent fluid retention, avoid standing for long periods of time, and rest with your legs up. Avoid foods high in sodium.

## Flutters

These symptoms precede quickening, or perception of fetal movement, by a few weeks. These sensations are typically described as bubbles, or butterflies, that are felt intermittently within the lower abdomen.

## Folic Acid

If you are contemplating a pregnancy, you should eat a balanced diet that is rich in folic acid, or take a prenatal vitamin supplement each day. Folic acid is a vitamin that is essential for the proper development of the fetus's nervous system, including the brain and the spinal cord. The recommended amount of folic acid is 400 to 800 micrograms daily for three or more months prior to conception and during pregnancy.

## Follicle

A follicle is a small sac, or cavity, composed of cells—for instance, the ovarian follicle produces the egg or ovum.

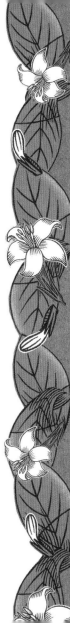

## Forceps

Forceps are metal instruments that look like two big spoons locked together. Forceps are used on certain occasions to assist with the delivery of your baby.

## Frequent Urination

This urge is due to the pressure caused by the growing uterus upon the bladder in early pregnancy, and later on by the pressure caused by the growing fetus. Avoid drinking too much in the evening so you can sleep through the night. Frequent urination, especially of sudden onset and when accompanied by burning, may be due to a bladder infection, in which case you should see your health-care provider.

## Fundal Height

As your pregnancy progresses, your uterus expands. During each visit to your health-care provider, beginning after the 12th week, your fundal height will be measured to evaluate the size of your uterus. Fundal height is measured from the top of the pubic bone to the top of the rounded uterus or fundus. If there is any question about fetal growth, whether it is growing fast or lagging, a sonogram can be ordered. The fundal height reaches the symphysis pubis by the 12th week, is midway between the symphysis pubis and the umbilicus by the 16th week, at the umbilicus by the 20th week, and just below the rib cage by term.

## Genetic Testing

Genetic testing is advised for women with a family history of genetic defects, or those age 35 or older.

## Girl

The cute newborn baby with "indoor plumbing."

## Glucola

Glucola is a special soda-like sugar solution used for the glucose screen.

## Glucose Screen

A glucose screen may be performed around your 24th to 28th week to rule out diabetes. You will be asked to drink glucola, and your blood will be drawn one hour later to check its sugar level.

## Glucose Tolerance Test

If your glucose screen is abnormal, you will be required to undergo a three-hour glucose tolerance test. If these test results are also abnormal, you will be diagnosed with gestational diabetes.

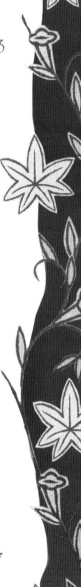

## Gonorrhea

This is an acute disease of the lining (epithelium) of the urethra, cervix, and rectum, transmitted by direct sexual contact. It can be cured with antibiotics. Symptoms usually appear within 2 to 14 days after contact among men, and within 7 to 21 days after contact among women. Men can experience painful urination and a whitish discharge from the penis, rectum, and eyes; the throat may also be infected. Some infected men have no symptoms. Women may have a whitish, yellowish, or greenish vaginal or anal discharge, but 80 percent of infected women have no symptoms. Without treatment, gonorrhea can cause pelvic inflammatory disease, sterility, blindness, arthritis, and heart disease. Gonorrhea can also be passed to newborn babies during childbirth. All pregnant women are tested for gonorrhea during their first prenatal visit.

## Grantly Dick-Read Method

This childbirth method consists of three components:

1. The teaching of the anatomy and physiology of childbirth to dispel the notion that childbirth must be painful.
2. The teaching of physical conditioning, relaxation techniques, and breathing exercises.
3. Having complete faith in your birth attendant.

## Group B Strep

A pregnant mother is checked for Group B Strep between her 34th and 36th week. Group B Strep has been associated with severe neonatal infection. Secretions are sampled from the outer vagina and the rectum, and a culture is done. If the culture is positive, the mother will be treated with antibiotics during labor.

## Guided Imagery

The power of the mind can be used to evoke a positive physical response during guided use of the imagination. This can reduce stress, slow your heart rate, stimulate your immune system, and reduce pain. I use this method in my practice to help patients relieve anxiety, stress, and nausea throughout pregnancy.

## Hair

Your hair might get thicker *during* your pregnancy, but there can be a tendency to *lose* hair during the two to four months following delivery. Do not panic; your hair will grow in within 6 to 12 months.

## Headache

Headache is one of the most common types of pain associated with pregnancy. Most headaches are tension headaches, also known as muscle contraction headaches, and may be relieved with acetaminophen. Women with a history of migraines may continue to experience these headaches during their pregnancy. Severe and constant headaches may be a sign of pre-eclampsia and should immediately be reported to your health-care provider.

## Health-Care Provider

The person who is responsible for your medical care during your pregnancy. This individual may be an obstetrician, family doctor, nurse practitioner, physician assistant, nurse-midwife, or someone else.

## Heartbeat

The fetus's heart begins to beat around the 25th day of gestation. It can be detected by ultrasound as early as five to six weeks of gestation, and heard with a doppler, or hand-held soundwave stethoscope, at about nine to ten weeks of gestation. One of the greatest moments in a woman's pregnancy can be hearing her baby's heartbeat for the first time. It can bring tears and laughter simultaneously. The heartbeat has been described as sounding like a choo-choo train or galloping horse.

## Heartburn

Increased progesterone levels during pregnancy relax the muscles of the esophageal sphincter, and the enlarged uterus pushes the stomach and esophagus upward. The esophagus is the tube leading from your mouth to your stomach. Heartburn is the result of the backup of stomach acid into the esophagus, resulting in a burning pain felt behind the breastbone.

Heartburn may sometimes be accompanied by an unpleasant taste in the mouth, or belching. To prevent heartburn:

* Use antacids, but avoid taking too much since this may decrease the absorption of iron. Liquid antacids are more effective because they coat the esophagus.

- Raise the foot of your bed to prevent reflux.
- Chew gum for 30 minutes after a meal to help stimulate the production of saliva, which neutralizes stomach acid and washes out the esophagus. But don't chew gum if you have flatulence.
- Drink chamomile tea.
- Avoid spicy foods, citrus fruits, and overeating.
- Eat several small meals throughout the day.
- Wait two hours after eating to exercise or lie down.

## Hemoglobin

Hemoglobin is the iron-containing pigment of your red blood cells. A protein compound in the blood, it carries oxygen from the lungs to the body tissues.

## Hemorrhage

Heavy bleeding.

## Hemorrhoids

These are varicose veins of the rectum. When the hemorrhoidal veins within the rectum become enlarged and recede into the canal, they are called hemorrhoids. Over time, these veins can hang outside the anus. Constipation, marked by straining during defecation, is one of the causes of hemorrhoids. The

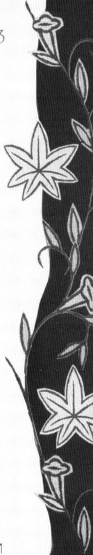

most common symptoms are bleeding and rectal pain, soreness, and itching around the anus. To help prevent constipation, drink six to eight glasses of fluids per day, and eat a fiber-rich diet. You may wish to take fiber supplements such as Metamucil. Avoid standing for long periods of time. For painful hemorrhoids, five-minute sitz baths, three to four times a day, can ease your discomfort. Ice packs, warm baths, and acupuncture have also been found to be helpful. Talk to your health-care provider about suppositories or stool softeners, and avoid taking laxatives.

## Hepatitis B

Hepatitis B is a highly contagious type of liver inflammation caused by a viral infection. It is contracted through contact with infected human blood or people with sexually transmitted diseases. About one in 250 Americans is a chronic carrier. Symptoms may appear between six weeks and six months from initial contact, and include nausea and vomiting, abdominal pain, loss of appetite, and yellowing of the skin and the whites of the eyes.

During your first prenatal visit, a blood test will be performed to determine if you are immune to Hepatitis B. If your blood test is positive, your newborn infant will be treated with the hepatitis B immune globulin vaccine. If you work in a health-care environment or you are often in contact with blood or blood products, you should receive the hepatitis B immune globulin vaccine to prevent infection before getting pregnant.

## Hepatitis C

About four million Americans have hepatitis C, a chronic liver infection that can lead to cirrhosis of the liver and the eventual need for a liver transplant. Five percent of cases are transmitted from the mother to the infant. You should be tested for hepatitis C if you had a blood transfusion prior to 1992.

## Herbs

Because some herbs and tinctures or their combination with prescription drugs may be detrimental to your health and to the health of your fetus, you need to follow the recommendations of a competent and trusted health-care provider. Do not self-prescribe! However, herbal teas such as mint, ginger, and chamomile are safe.

## Herpes (genital)

Herpes is an inflammatory viral infection that is transmitted sexually and causes eruptions and ulcers of the skin. Symptoms usually appear within 2 to 20 days of contact with a person infected with the virus. In some cases, the first eruption may not appear until months or years after contact. The symptoms may be so mild—just slight discomfort—that a person doesn't realize an eruption is occurring and may unknowingly infect a sexual partner. Generally, symptoms consist of itching, pain in the genital area (or mouth), and painful blisters and ulcerations. Also, a lack of symptoms does not mean that you aren't contagious; a person may infect a partner in the complete absence of symptoms.

Once you are infected, the herpes virus remains inactive in the nerve roots and can recur at any time. Keeping the area clean and dry and avoiding sexual contact during an eruption will prevent transmission of the virus. There is no cure for genital herpes, but antiviral medications can hasten the healing process after an eruption and prevent recurrences.

A pregnant woman may pass the infection to her newborn if the baby comes into contact with an infected area. If labor begins while the disease is active, a cesarean section will most likely be performed.

## High Blood Pressure

High blood pressure, or hypertension, occurs when blood flows too forcefully through the blood vessels, potentially causing damage to the vessel walls, which may cause a heart attack, stroke, or kidney failure. High blood pressure is also one indication of toxemia. Women with hypertension have a higher likelihood of developing pre-eclampsia.

## HIV (Human Immunodeficiency Virus)

HIV, regarded as responsible for the development of AIDS, can be transmitted sexually, during transfusion of infected blood, or from the mother to the fetus. HIV screening is recommended for all pregnant women. If a woman is HIV positive, drug treatment can reduce the risk of transmission to her fetus by two-thirds. Delivery by cesarean section has been demonstrated to reduce the transmission of HIV to the baby. Since HIV can also be transmitted through breast milk, an infected mother should not breast-feed.

## Home Birth

A home birth is, obviously, when the baby is born at home, often with a midwife in attendance. Home births should be chosen by women with no known medical risks. Because your life and the life of your baby is in her hands, choose your midwife carefully, check her references, and also make arrangements with a local obstetrician and a hospital in case of an emergency.

## Home Pregnancy Test

Readily available and accurate, the outcome of such a test should be confirmed at your health-care provider's office.

## Hospital Birth

You and your health-care provider should agree upon the hospital where your delivery will take place. You may wish to visit the various hospitals where your health-care provider delivers and evaluate the types of birthing environments available prior to making your decision. You may be limited to hospitals that your health-care provider is affiliated with, as well as those that are covered by your health insurance. Some factors to keep in mind during your evaluation are: convenience, amenities, availability of a neonatal unit, and the type of birthing room available.

You should go to the hospital if and when:

* your contractions are regular (every two to three minutes for one to two hours for a first baby, and one hour for subsequent deliveries);

* you suspect your membranes have ruptured; and/or

* vaginal bleeding occurs.

Today in the United States, after a vaginal birth without complications, the normal stay is two days. Following a cesarean section, you may stay up to four days.

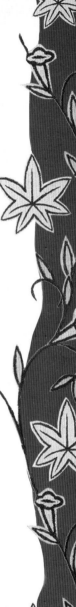

## Human Chorionic Gonadotropin (HCG)

This is a hormone that is produced by the corpus luteum within a week of conception; levels typically double in value every two to three days and continue to rise throughout your pregnancy. This hormone is what is detected by a pregnancy test.

## Hydramnios

A condition that occurs during the later stages of pregnancy when there is an excessive amount of amniotic fluid in the amniotic sac. This condition can put the mother at risk for premature labor. It is common with twin pregnancies and among women with pre-eclampsia.

## Hydrotherapy

You might like to try using this type of steam therapy to help break up congestion caused by the common cold or flu. Boil water in a pot, add one to two tablespoons of mint leaves and a few drops of wintergreen or eucalyptus oil, remove from the heat source, and carefully inhale the steam so as not to burn yourself.

## Hyperemesis Gravidarum

This is a severe form of nausea and vomiting, associated with weight loss, ketonemia, electrolyte imbalance, dehydration, and kidney and liver damage if prolonged. Hospitalization is often necessary. Hyperemesis gravidarum affects 1 to 2 percent of all pregnancies.

## Hypertension

Also referred to as high blood pressure.

## Hypnosis

Hypnosis is when someone conducts hypnotherapy on you. Self-hypnosis can be learned and can be helpful in alleviating pain during labor.

## Hypnotherapy

Hypnotherapy is the induction of a willing subject into a state of focused concentration, described as neither wakefulness nor sleep, and during which the subject is open and responsive to suggestion.

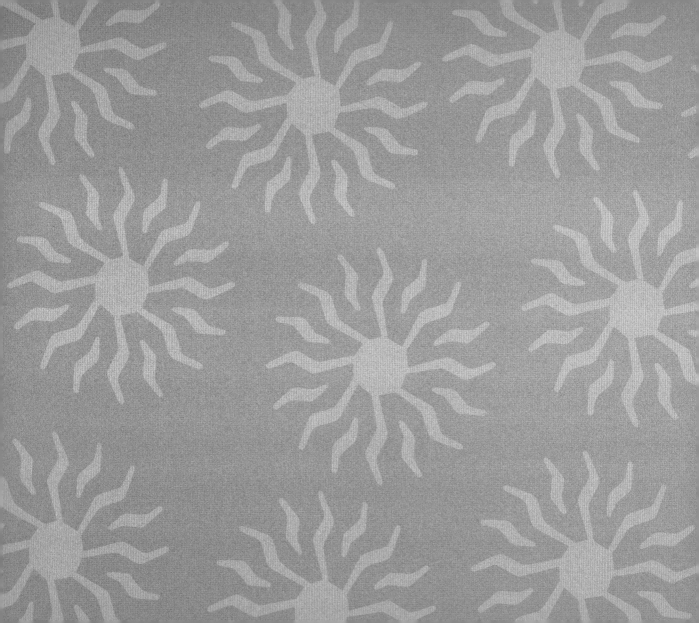

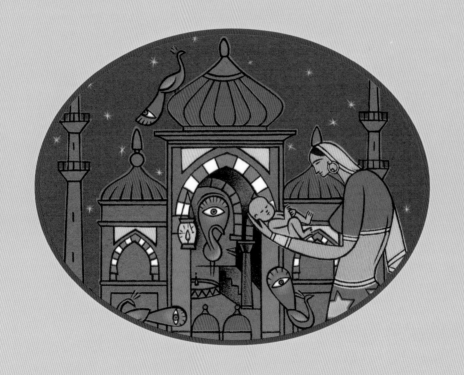

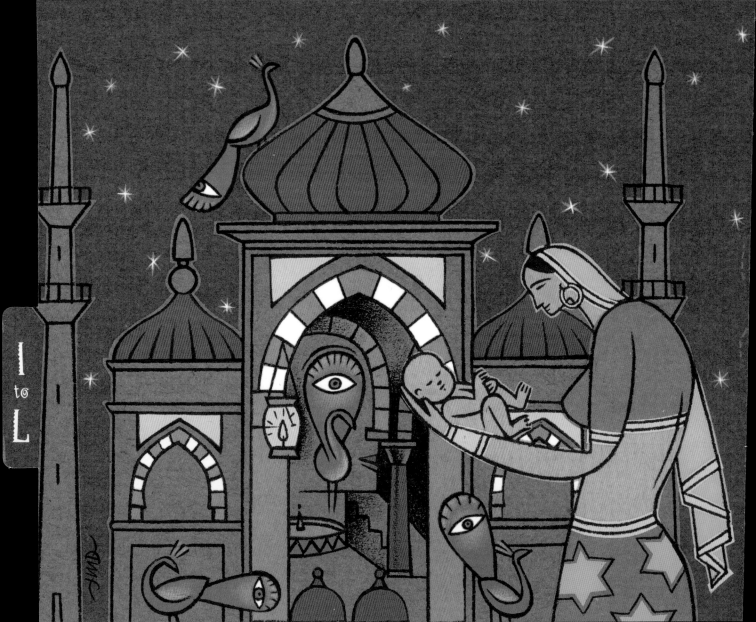

## Ibuprofen

Ibuprofen (Nuprin, Motrin, Aleve, and Advil) should not be taken during pregnancy. Use of ibuprofen can result in thinning of the blood and may cause heart disease in the newborn.

## Ice Packs

Ice packs may be used to reduce inflammation and swelling. Ice packs are available commercially, you can make your own by placing ice chips in a plastic bag, or you may use a bag of frozen peas (I prefer sweet peas). Ice packs should be applied for 20 minutes, every 4 hours, for the first 24 hours after an episiotomy, and for 24 to 36 hours for hemorrhoids.

## Immunization

Immunization is the process of activating the body's immune response against a specific disease, usually with an inoculation.

## Implantation

Implantation occurs when a fertilized egg attaches itself to the uterine wall.

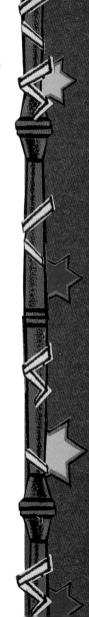

## Incomplete Abortion

When a spontaneous abortion occurs and only part of the product of conception is expelled, this is referred to as an incomplete abortion. A dilation and curettage (D&C) is necessary to remove the remaining tissue.

## Incontinence

Common among pregnant women, urinary incontinence is the involuntary loss of bladder control or an inability to predict when and where urination will occur. It can occur after childbirth or during the menopausal years. To prevent incontinence, Kegel exercises can be helpful. Constipation should be avoided, and the bladder should be emptied often.

## Induction of Labor

Labor may have to be induced when the benefits of delivery outweigh those of continuing the pregnancy.

## Infertility

As a woman ages, a decline in fertility, or the ability to become pregnant, occurs. This decline begins during a woman's early 30s, when she begins to ovulate less frequently. Infertility has been formally defined as the inability to conceive after 12 to 18 months of regular intercourse without birth control. Forty percent of infertility is due to a female factor, another 40 percent to a male factor. About 20 percent of infertile

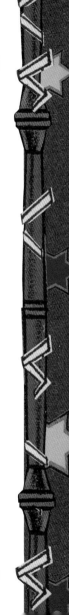

couples have no known factor, and about 80 percent of couples who are actively trying to conceive tend to succeed within a year. Advanced reproductive techniques have allowed many couples with challenging problems to have children. These techniques include: in vitro fertilization (IVF), gamete intrafallopian transfer (GIFT), and zygote intrafallopian transfer (ZIFT).

## Inflammation

Inflammation is a reddening and swelling of body tissue as a reaction to infection or cellular injury.

## Insomnia

Pregnant women have difficulty sleeping, especially during the last trimester, often because it is a struggle to find a comfortable position. You may also be kept awake by an active, kicking baby; sweating; hot flashes caused by increased blood supply, or because of frequent urination due to the pressure of your uterus on your bladder. Try to avoid lying on your back; you'll be more comfortable lying on your side, with pillows to support your upper thighs and abdomen.

## Insurance

Make sure you have health insurance before planning to conceive. Pregnancy is viewed as a preexisting condition by many insurance carriers, and you may find that you are unable to purchase coverage. A pregnancy without health insurance can be a costly endeavor.

## Internal Fetal Monitoring

During this procedure, an electrode is inserted through your vagina, cervix, and into the uterus, and applied to the baby's scalp to measure the heart rate. Your contractions may also be monitored by inserting a pressure catheter—a long, thin tube—in the same manner. Each device is attached to a monitor that allows your provider to print out the information gathered.

## Intrauterine Growth Retardation (IUGR)

This condition complicates about 3 to 7 percent of all pregnancies. When the fetus does not grow as expected, it may have an increased risk for complications during labor and after birth. If your health-care provider suspects that you have this condition, the fetus will be followed closely, and in some cases, labor may be induced before term.

## Intrauterine Insemination

Intrauterine insemination is a procedure whereby washed sperm are injected into the uterus of an infertile woman at the time of her ovulation.

## Intravenous Line

An intravenous line may be used to deliver fluids or medications during your labor and delivery. Plastic tubing, attached to a needle, is inserted into a vein in your arm and connected to a bag of liquid. If you'd like more freedom of movement, you may be able to request that a heparin lock be added to your IV.

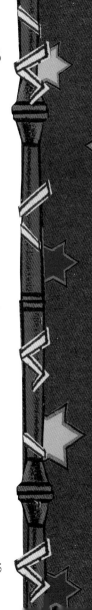

## In Vitro Fertilization

During in vitro fertilization, many eggs are matured with fertility drugs, and then are harvested and fertilized outside of the womb. The fertilized embryos are then returned to the uterine cavity. Multiple births may ensue. *In vitro* literally means "in glass." Fertilization is accomplished in a test tube; hence, the term "test tube baby." In vitro fertilization is performed when the Fallopian tubes are blocked, if the ovaries are damaged, or when an egg is donated by another woman.

## Iron Supplements

If you are anemic, your health-care provider will prescribe iron supplements. The iron may cause constipation and dark discoloration of the stools. Drink at least eight, 8-ounce glasses of fluids per day, and eat a high-fiber diet.

## Itching

Itching can be the result of irritated or stretched skin, due to increased estrogen levels. Itching tends to be more pronounced on the abdomen and breasts. Relief can be obtained by avoiding soap and perfumed products and by using moisturizing creams and vitamin E oil.

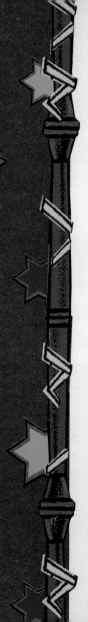

## Jacuzzi

Spas, saunas, Jacuzzis, whirlpools, hot tubs, and hot baths should be avoided during your pregnancy, since excessively high temperatures in the developing embryo may be associated with damage to the nervous system. Lukewarm baths, which are soothing and relaxing, are permitted.

## Jaundice

All newborn babies are born with some degree of jaundice because the liver cannot process bilirubin, a substance formed by the breakdown of hemoglobin. Fifty percent of all newborns develop a yellowish tinge by the second to fifth day after birth, which will usually clear up within ten days. For persistent or severe jaundice, the newborn may be admitted to the nursery for phototherapy, where your baby is exposed to special lights.

## Kegel Exercises

Dr. Arnold Kegel invented specific pelvic-floor exercises, also known as Kegel exercises, during the 1950s. These exercises involve contracting the muscles that regulate and stop your urine flow. To locate these muscles, try to stop your urine flow the next time you urinate. To perform these exercises, tighten your muscles without lifting your buttocks, and hold for 10 to 15 seconds, then release. In the beginning, you may have to do them for a shorter period of time, then increase as your muscles become stronger. Rest for at least ten seconds between each contraction, and repeat 10 to 15 times, three to five times a day, or as often as you can while driving or watching television. Repetition is important! Make sure that each contraction is as hard as you can manage. It is also a good habit to contract these muscles prior to coughing, sneezing, or nose-blowing.

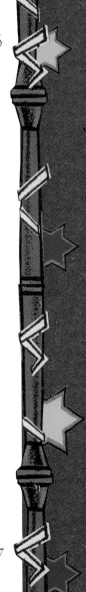

During the Kegel exercises, be aware of using your stomach, buttocks, or leg muscles. While squeezing your muscles, place your hand on your abdomen. If you feel it move, you are using your abdominal muscles, too. Your goal is to isolate and use only your pelvic muscles. Kegel exercises should be done regularly during and after pregnancy. Performing Kegel exercises regularly can help to decrease incontinence and increase muscle strength.

## Kick Count

A kick count is an assessment of daily fetal movements, including rolls, flutters, or kicks. A healthy fetus is supposed to be moving around, especially during the early evening hours. Beginning at 28 weeks, you can do this count while resting comfortably, reading, or watching TV. The perception of ten distinct movements in a period of up to two hours is considered reassuring. If your baby is not moving as usual, contact your health-care provider immediately.

## Kidney Infection

If left untreated, a bladder infection may lead to a kidney infection, or pyelonephritis. Symptoms include fever, back pain, and sometimes nausea and vomiting. If left untreated, it can lead to premature labor. A kidney infection in a pregnant woman is usually treated in the hospital with intravenous antibiotics.

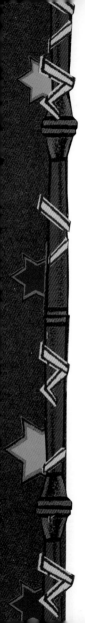

## Labor

Labor marks the end of your pregnancy. Most women experience labor without complications. You are in labor when your contractions are:

* regular and get closer together;

* steadily increase in strength;

* continuous, in spite of movement; and

* usually felt in your back, and then move to your front.

Labor is divided into three stages. The first stage, dilatation, is achieved when your cervix is completely dilated and may last as long as 6 to 18 hours for your first pregnancy, and 3 to 10 hours for subsequent births. The second stage, expulsion, begins with pushing and ends with the delivery of the baby. Pushing can last from 30 minutes to three hours for your first baby, and from 30 minutes to one hour for subsequent births. During this stage, your contractions will come more rapidly, are harder, and may last from 30 to 60 seconds. The third stage ends with the delivery of the placenta and may last from 5 to 20 minutes.

## Lactation

Lactation is the production and release of milk from your breasts after you have given birth.

## Lamaze Method

Childbirth classes that stress relaxation and breathing techniques for each stage of labor are known as the Lamaze method.

## Last Menstrual Period (LMP)

Since it is impossible to define when conception occurs, the first day of the last menstrual period is considered to be the official beginning of your pregnancy.

## Late Deceleration

Deceleration, or slowing of the fetal heart rate, may occur well after a contraction is under way and is indicative of fetal distress.

## Leboyer Method

With the Leboyer method, your baby will be delivered in a serene atmosphere with dim light. The umbilical cord will be clamped only after it has stopped pulsating. The baby will be given a warm bath after birth.

## Leg Cramps

Leg cramps are frequent during pregnancy, are most common during the last three months, and usually occur while you are lying down. The cause is unknown.

To prevent leg cramps, try this exercise: Face a wall standing three feet away, and place the palms of both your hands upward against the wall. Step forward with your left foot. Bend your left leg while keeping your feet flat on the floor and your toes pointed ahead. While keeping your back straight, bend forward and hold the position for five seconds. You will feel your calf muscles stretch. Repeat with the right leg. To relieve leg cramps, walk slowly until they subside. Flex your feet by pushing your heels away from you. Cramps can also be relieved with gentle massage.

## Libido

Sex drive, or sexual desire, may decrease during your pregnancy. Sexual desire can also vary from trimester to trimester and from woman to woman. If you are unable to have intercourse, try holding hands, kissing, and massage to help your partner feel less rejected. Your libido may also decrease after childbirth. This is due in part to natural hormone changes and fatigue, which decreases vaginal lubrication, especially if you are breast-feeding. For vaginal dryness, try lubricants or vitamin E oil.

## Lightening

Lightening is a term referring to the changing position of the baby a few hours to a few weeks before your actual labor begins. It occurs when your baby drops and its head settles into the birth canal before the onset of labor.

100

## Lochia

Lochia is postpartum uterine discharge consisting of blood flow that lasts for several hours after child-birth, which then diminishes to a reddish-brown discharge that lasts through the fourth or fifth postpartum day. Thereafter, there is a mucoid, reddish to pinkish discharge that lasts for up to four to six weeks and is occasionally malodorous. Infrequently, you may experience a transient period of bleeding, sometimes heavy. If the bleeding does not subside within two hours, call your health-care provider to be evaluated for possible retention of placental tissue.

## Low Birth Weight

When a newborn weighs less than five and a half pounds, it is considered to be of low birth weight. Low birth weight may be due to conditions such as hypertension, smoking, and prematurity.

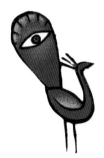

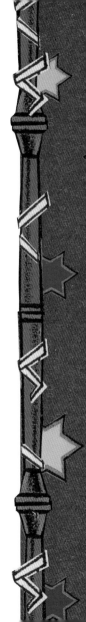

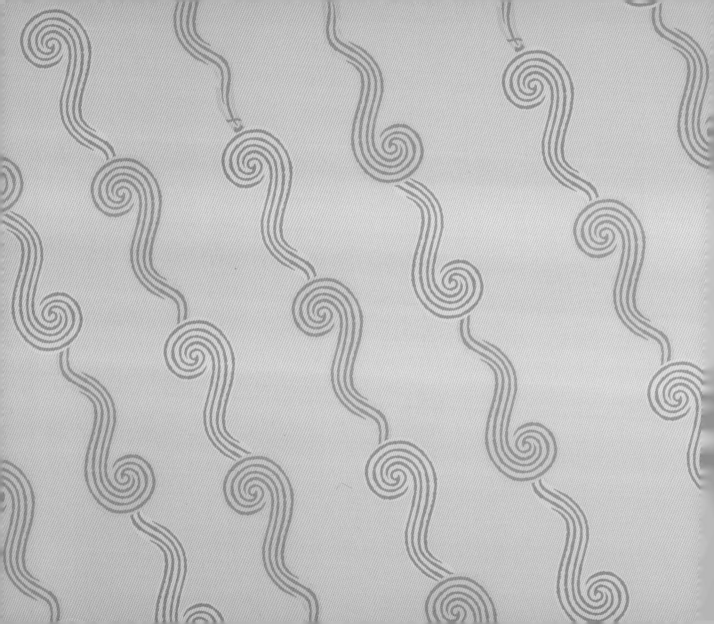

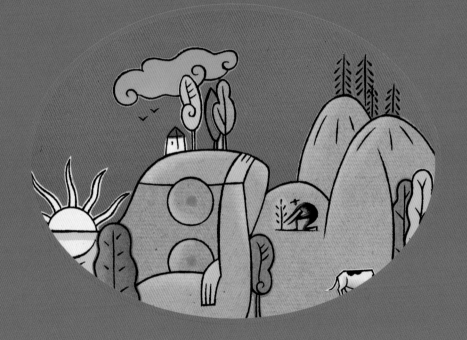

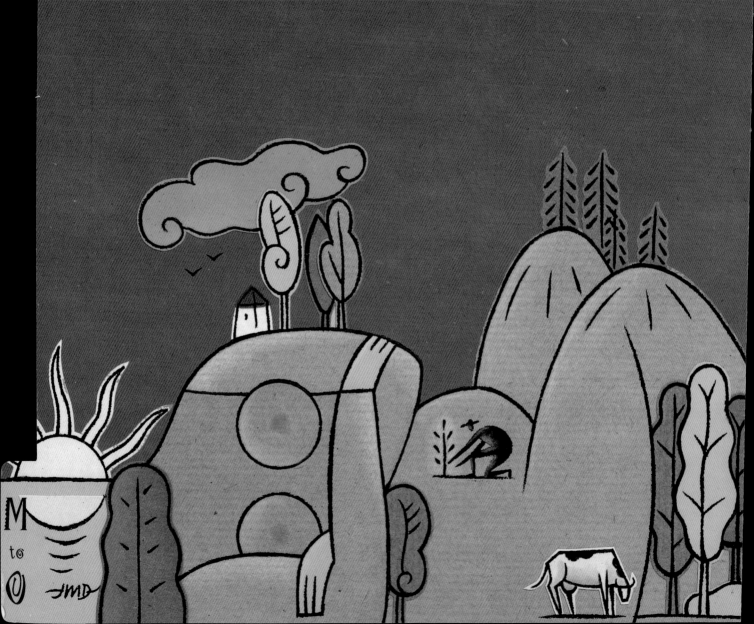

## Malpresentation

Among approximately 5 percent of all labors, the fetus does not come out head first. Other presentations include:

* breech presentation—3 to 4 percent of all births;
* face presentation—one in 500 births; and
* brow presentation—one in 1,500 births.

## Massage

Massage is the systemic manipulation of soft tissue with hand strokes and occasional static pressure. It has been demonstrated that physical touch increases the rate of healing, enhances the immune system, and stimulates the body to release hormones, called endorphins, which are responsible for a feeling of well-being. Massage therapy can also be used to alleviate depression, headaches, insomnia, stress, anxiety, and tension. Massage can be a great way to relieve labor pain, muscle spasms, leg cramps, headaches, varicose veins, and swelling; it can also increase circulation.

I recommend careful light massage for pregnant women to relieve symptoms, and also as a natural way to stay physically and emotionally close with their partners.

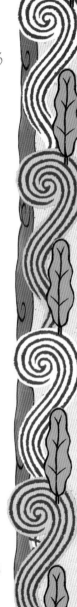

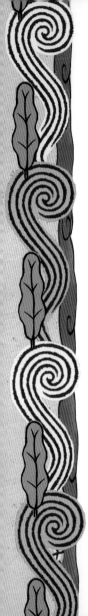

## Mastitis

Mastitis is an inflammatory process of the breast. It is especially common among women who are breast-feeding. Mastitis is associated with tenderness and redness of the skin and can easily be treated with antibiotics. Infrequently an abscess forms, which requires surgical drainage.

## Meconium

A greenish-black mucuslike substance present in the intestines of a fetus is called meconium. In the event of fetal distress, the fetus may have its first bowel movement. This is a common problem in postterm pregnancies and can be dangerous if swallowed by the fetus, thereby blocking its airway passages.

## Medications

During the pre-conceptual period, and during your pregnancy, prescription medications should be used with care. In some cases, the benefits of their use may outweigh the possible risks during pregnancy. Do not use over-the-counter drugs without prior consultation with your health-care provider.

## Meditation

Meditation is a state of quiet contemplation. In simple meditation, a person sits quietly and focuses her mind on a single thought. In mindful meditation, a person sits quietly and simply witnesses whatever goes through her mind, without reaction. Studies have demonstrated that meditation causes a generalized reduc-

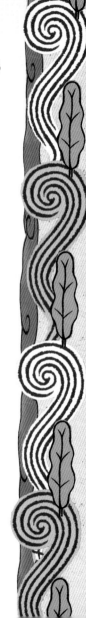

tion in heart rate and respiration rate, decreases cortisol (a major stress hormone) and pulse rate, and increases alpha brain waves associated with relaxation. A recent study demonstrated that meditating for 20 minutes, twice a day, can decrease blood pressure significantly. Meditation can also be used to relieve stress and panic disorders and can be a helpful technique to relieve pain and anxiety during labor.

## Menstrual Cycle

Your menstrual cycle is approximately a four-week period during which one of your ovaries produces an egg for fertilization, your body sheds the unfertilized egg along with the lining of your uterus (menstruation), and your ovaries again prepare to produce an egg.

## Midwife

A midwife has special training to take care of a woman during pregnancy, labor, and delivery. Midwives can attend deliveries at home, birthing centers, and hospitals. During deliveries that are attended by midwives, laboring women typically require less pain medication, receive fewer episiotomies, and are less likely to deliver by cesarean section. Home births by a midwife should be chosen only by women who have no known medical risks. Because your life and the life of your baby is in her hands, choose your midwife carefully, check her references, and also make arrangements with a local obstetrician and a hospital in case of an emergency.

## Miscarriage

When the loss of the fetus occurs before the 28th week of pregnancy, this is referred to as a miscarriage. Eighty percent of all miscarriages are caused by abnormalities in the developing embryo. Miscarriage,

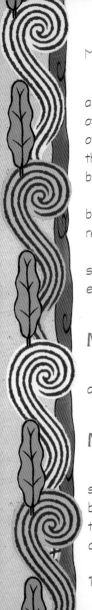

also known as spontaneous abortion, occurs in as many as 25 to 35 percent of all pregnancies, and most of them during the first 12 weeks of pregnancy. In fact, most miscarriages occur within the first few weeks of pregnancy, often before a woman realizes that she is pregnant. The cause is unknown, but it is believed that most miscarriages occur naturally when the embryo develops poorly and has characteristics incompatible with life.

After a miscarriage, it is usually recommended that you wait at least three normal menstrual cycles before attempting the next pregnancy in order to increase your chances of having a healthy baby. Testing is recommended only after a woman has experienced three spontaneous abortions during the early trimesters.

The loss of a pregnancy at any stage can be devastating to a woman and her family, causing immense sadness and profound distress. Participation in a support group with other women who have had a similar experience, or one-on-one counseling, can be helpful during this time.

## Molar Pregnancy

A molar pregnancy is an abnormal pregnancy where fertilization does not result in a healthy embryo. What does occur is a tumor, resembling a cluster of grapes, which needs to be removed with a dilation and curettage (D&C).

## Morning Sickness

Welcome to the club! Morning sickness occurs in 60 to 70 percent of all pregnancies, consisting of symptoms including nausea, vomiting and retching, and intolerance to specific foods. Morning sickness may be due in part to the increase of circulating hormones, and is most severe during the first 12 weeks of gestation. It may be comforting to learn that, in my experience, women who suffer from morning sickness typically have a very small chance of miscarrying.

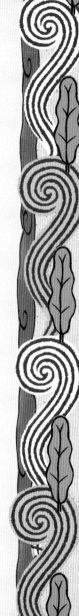

## Mother

You will become a mother after giving birth to a baby. You are now entitled to receive special treatment on Mother's Day!

## Mucous Plug

The mucous glands of the cervix create a mucous plug that seals the cervical opening. About 24 hours before labor begins, the mucous plug that has guarded the entrance of the cervix may break loose. Sometimes it may be mixed with blood; hence, the name "bloody show."

## Multipara

A woman who has had a previous birth.

## Multiple Births

Most babies from multiple births are born healthy, but there is an increased risk of premature labor, anemia, and high blood pressure in the mother, as well as low birth weight in the babies. Multiple births that occur naturally are more common among black women than white women. The incidence of multiple births is on the increase due to the use of fertility drugs.

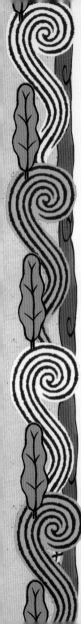

## Natural Childbirth

Women have been having natural childbirth for millions of years. When a woman decides to forgo any medical intervention to relieve pain during labor, this is considered natural childbirth. Pain relief can be accomplished by natural methods, such as acupressure, warm baths, breathing techniques, yoga, and hot showers.

## Nausea

This frequent and uncomfortable symptom can be brought on by familiar smells or strong smells, and may range from mild to severe. It is worse on an empty stomach. Nausea and vomiting usually occur among 70 percent of all pregnancies. The typical onset is between four to eight weeks, continuing through the 14th to 16th week. In rare instances, nausea may last through your second trimester. Some home remedies for nausea include teas from nutmeg, peppermint, lemon balm, cinnamon, and ginger. You might also try wearing an acupressure wristband, easily purchased in drugstores. Other comfort recommendations are:

* Avoid an empty stomach by ingesting frequent small snacks or mini meals throughout the day.
* Drink plenty of fluids.
* Avoid foods that trigger nausea.
* Arise from bed slowly in the morning.
* Avoid very hot or very cold beverages.
* Avoid fried, greasy, and spicy foods.

## Neonatologist

A neonatologist is a specialist in the care of premature newborns, or newborns who suffered complications during labor and delivery.

## Neural Tube Defects

Neural tube defects are the result of the abnormal development of the fetal brain and/or spinal cord.

## Newborn

The newborn is the gift you receive at the end of your pregnancy. "Average" babies weigh approximately 7 lbs., 7oz., and measure 20 inches in length.

## Newborn Parenting Courses

Newborn parenting courses are a must for every new parent. While pregnancy is a natural occurrence, parenting skills must be learned.

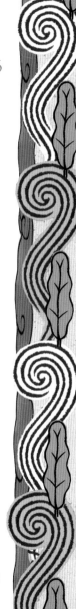

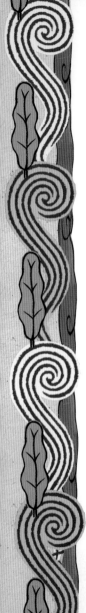

## Nipple Discharge

A nipple discharge other than milk does not usually indicate breast cancer. A yellowish discharge can be present as early as the first trimester of pregnancy. Fibrocystic changes may cause a green or brown fluid leaking from the nipple. Occasionally, a small growth may be discovered within the milk duct, usually near the nipple; this can cause a bloody nipple discharge. These tumors should be removed surgically. All breast discharges should be evaluated by a health-care provider.

## Non-Stress Test

A non-stress test is performed in your doctor's office or hospital setting and is used to evaluate fetal well-being. A fetal monitor is connected to a belt strapped around the pregnant woman's abdomen, and the fetal heartbeat is registered. A healthy fetus's heart rate increases with fetal movements.

## Nosebleed

During your pregnancy, there is an increase in blood supply that may cause a stuffy nose and, occasionally, a nosebleed. Try to avoid excessively dry rooms, and during the winter months, use a humidifier to keep the air moist. Avoid dry, dusty environments, and do not use nasal sprays.

## Nullipara

A woman who has not yet given birth.

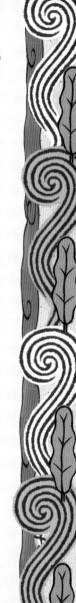

## Nurse Practitioner

A nurse practitioner is a nurse with an advanced degree in a certain area of medicine who can provide basic primary care under the supervision of a physician.

## Nursery

The newborn's special space should include at least a crib, chair, and changing table in addition to all baby supplies. Decorating cheerfully will lift spirits, including yours, and stimulate your baby's interest and attention.

## Nutrition

A healthy diet is necessary for *your* health as well as that of your baby. Eat plenty of fresh fruits and vegetables; protein such as fish and lean meats; dairy products that are rich in calcium; beans, eggs, whole grains or enriched breads; and dried fruits. Eggs, liver, kidneys, and green leafy vegetables are rich in iron and will help you avoid anemia. Drink six to eight glasses of liquid daily—including soups, fruit juices, and other beverages in addition to water.

## Obstetrician-Gynecologist

This is a medical doctor who specializes in the reproductive health of women. Check with your obstetrician's policy regarding natural labor, use of episiotomy, and pain relief.

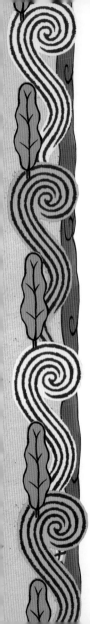

## Ovary

Your ovaries are located at the ends of each of your Fallopian tubes. They are oval-shaped glands, about the size of a walnut, and contain multiple follicles, or envelopes that hold eggs. The ovary is the site where the female sex hormones, estrogen and progesterone; and a small amount of the male hormone, testosterone, are produced.

## Overdue Baby

If your baby hasn't been delivered before your 42nd week, your baby is overdue. This occurs in approximately 10 percent of all pregnancies; between 3 and 12 percent of all pregnancies extend beyond the start of the 43rd week of gestation. A fetus is considered at increased risk after 42 weeks because the placenta may stop functioning. Your baby may also grow to be too large for a vaginal delivery. After 42 weeks, your doctor will perform tests to make sure that the fetus is healthy. These tests may include a non-stress test, biophysical profile, or a stress test. If there is any indication of distress, labor will be induced, and, in some cases, a C-section may be recommended.

## Overeating

Some pregnant women have the tendency to overeat because they believe that they are "eating for two." You do not need to eat twice as much as usual! A pregnant woman only needs about 300 to 500 extra calories per day. Overeating may lead to increased weight gain, which is associated with complications during labor and delivery. Overeating is also one cause of heartburn.

## Ovulation

The release of an egg from one of the ovaries.

## Ovum

The female egg.

## Oxytocin

Oxytocin is the natural hormone secreted by the brain's pituitary gland, which stimulates labor.

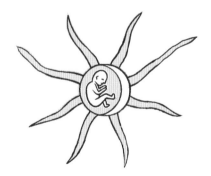

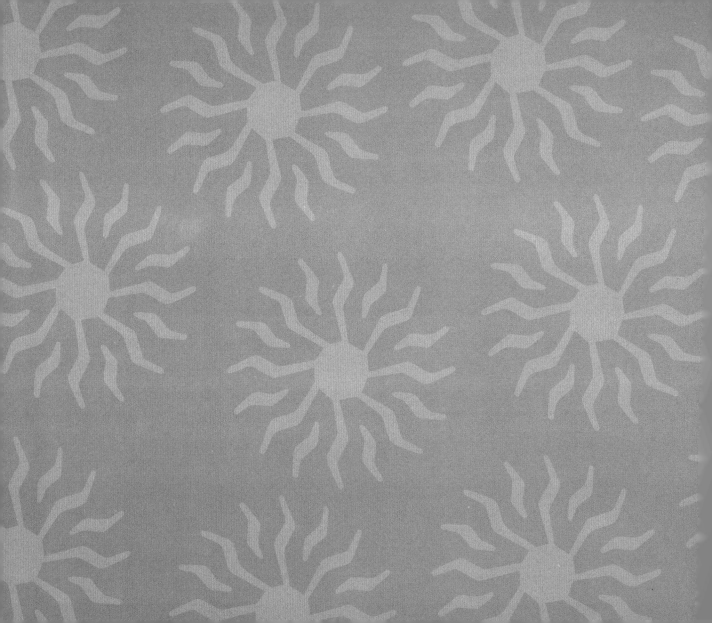

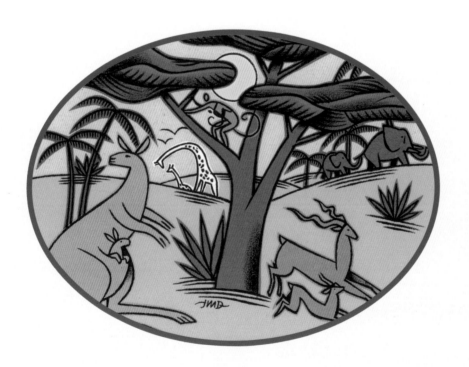

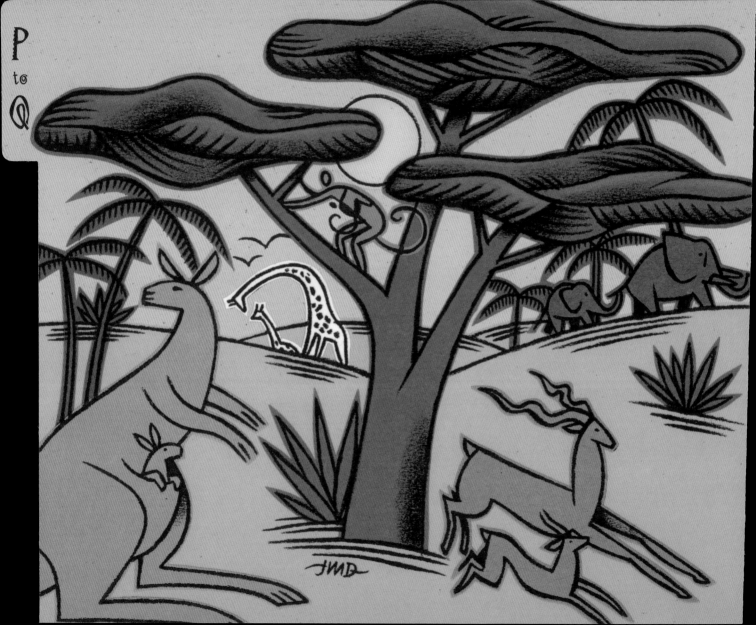

P
to
Q

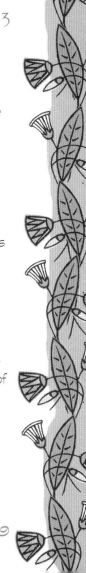

## Pain Relief

Instead of medication, pain relief can also be achieved via relaxation and breathing techniques, acupressure in the lower abdomen, use of a focal point at the peak of contractions, and working with the pain. One other way to relieve pain is by screaming. During labor, you can scream your heart out if it makes you feel better. Don't worry about it; most women in labor *do* scream.

Many women trying for a natural childbirth experience feel guilty if they request pain medication or anesthesia during labor and delivery. Different women deal with pain differently. You cannot hope to know how you'll handle the pain associated with labor and delivery if this is your first pregnancy. You have to believe that it is okay to request medication if you feel you need it.

The labor coach needs to understand when the woman wants pain relief. Personally, I have seen fetuses in distress because the woman was stressed with labor pains, and I have seen distress disappear when pain is relieved.

## Painful Urination

During pregnancy, painful urination is a sign of a bladder infection. After childbirth, because of the trauma to the perineum, urination can be painful when the acidic urine touches the area. You can relieve some of the pain by urinating in a warm bath or using a small squirt bottle to pour warm water over the area as you urinate on the toilet; sitz baths can also accelerate the healing of the perineum.

## Pap Smear

The Pap smear is a procedure where your medical provider takes a sample of cervical and vaginal cells in order to detect signs of precancerous conditions.

## Pediatrician

A pediatrician is a medical doctor who specializes in treating children.

## Pelvis

The bony ring that joins the spine and legs. Its central opening forms the walls of the birth canal.

## Percutaneous Umbilical Cord Blood Sampling (PUBS)

PUBS is performed after the 17th week of gestation, when required, and is used to detect fetal abnormalities.

## Perinatologist

A perinatologist is an obstetrician-gynecologist who is specialized and certified in maternal-fetal medicine. Your obstetrician will consult a perinatologist if there are complications that involve you, your fetus, or both. Chorionic villus sampling (CVS) and diagnostic amniocentesis for genetic purposes are performed by a perinatologist.

## Perineum

The perineum is the area between your vagina and anus that is cut during an episiotomy, prior to your baby's birth.

## Perms

Any hair treatment chemicals, including permanents and hair coloring, should be avoided during the pre-conceptual time and the first 12 weeks of pregnancy. In lieu of hair coloring, try highlights that do not involve the scalp, or use a natural hair coloring product made from henna. Also avoid hair salons where nails are manicured because of the strong chemical fumes.

## Physical Exam

During your first prenatal visit, your health-care provider will perform a complete physical exam. In addition, your pelvic bones will be evaluated for their adequacy for natural childbirth. A Pap smear and cervical cultures, to rule out any STDs, will also be performed. The health-care provider will evaluate the size of your uterus to confirm the EDC (estimated date of confinement)—the date your baby is expected to be born.

## Pitocin

Pitocin is a synthetic form of oxytocin, and it is used to induce or augment labor.

## Placenta

The placenta is a plate-shaped organ that links the blood supply of the woman to the fetus. It is attached to the fetus by the umbilical cord that carries oxygen and nutrients from the mother to the fetus.

In some cultures, the placenta is treated differently. My own grandmother strongly believed that after childbirth, the placenta should be buried in the mother's backyard to help a woman become infertile. (She was poor and had an irresponsible husband.) After the birth of her third child, she asked the midwife to bury the placenta. She remained sexually active for many years and never got pregnant again!

## Placenta Accreta

Placenta accreta is a condition where the placenta is attached to the uterus and is not easily removed after childbirth. This condition may cause severe postpartum hemorrhage, requiring an emergency hysterectomy.

## Placental Abruption

Also known as placenta abruptio, the placenta separates before birth; the cause is unknown. Women who smoke, use drugs, and have hypertension are at higher risk of placental abruption.

## Placenta Previa

Placenta previa, also called low-lying placenta, causes painless bleeding late in pregnancy, and can cause profuse bleeding during labor when the cervix starts to dilate. There are different degrees of previa, which include:

* marginal previa—when the placenta is located next to the cervical opening but does not touch or cover it;

* partial previa—when only a portion of the placenta obstructs the cervical opening; and

* complete previa—when the placenta completely blocks the cervical opening.

Placental location is usually confirmed by sonogram. If you have a placenta previa, you should abstain from intercourse and limit your physical activity.

## Postpartum

The time following the delivery of your baby.

## Postpartum Blues

Postpartum blues, or "baby blues," is a transient state of tearfulness, irritation, restlessness, and anxiety that occurs in up to 70 percent of new mothers. It usually begins around two to three days after childbirth, with the first flow of milk, and usually resolves by the tenth postpartum day. If it doesn't, it may develop into postpartum depression, requiring serious attention.

## Postpartum Checkup

Six weeks after childbirth you will be checked to see if everything has returned to normal. If you have a medical problem, or had a cesarean section, you may be asked to schedule an appointment sooner than six weeks with your health-care provider.

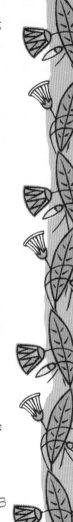

## Postpartum Depression

Postpartum depression occurs after childbirth, and in 10 percent of women. Symptoms may include excess sleepiness, weight loss, incapability of expressing emotion, and ambivalence toward the newborn baby. New parenthood can have a strong emotional impact on a woman. You may experience mood swings, from exhilaration to depression. During this period, your body is working hard to return to normal, even harder if you had a cesarean section. This healing, coupled with the physical toll of taking care of a demanding new baby, is sure to cause you some level of stress and/or depression. It can be helpful to understand that postpartum depression typically resolves itself spontaneously within ten weeks after birth, without professional intervention. If this condition interferes with your ability to function, see your health-care provider. You many require some counseling, and perhaps treatment with an antidepressant.

## Postpartum Hemorrhage

Excessive blood loss after a delivery is referred to as postpartum hemorrhage. The primary cause is that your uterine muscles do not contract firmly enough to control the bleeding produced when the placenta separates from the uterine wall. This condition can be corrected with intramuscular, or intravenous, medication to firm up the uterine muscles. Another cause is attributed to pieces of the placenta that remain inside the uterus and prevent it from contracting firmly. These remaining pieces have to be removed.

## Pre-Eclampsia

Pre-eclampsia is a complication of pregnancy that occurs among 7 percent of all pregnancies, and usually after the 35th week of pregnancy. Also called toxemia, it occurs more commonly among women having their first child. The cause is unknown. This is a dangerous condition that includes swelling, high blood pressure, and protein spilling into the urine. In severe cases, the mother may experience headache, blurred vision, "seeing spots," mental dullness, nausea, and vomiting. This condition can place the fetus and mother at risk. You should see your health-care provider right away if you experience any of the above symptoms. Women with high blood pressure have a greater likelihood of developing pre-eclampsia.

## Premature Baby

This is a baby that is delivered before the 37th week of pregnancy. Some may require a prolonged hospital stay and the care of a neonatologist.

## Premature Labor

When your labor occurs before your 37th week of pregnancy, it's considered premature. Premature births occur among 10 percent of all pregnancies and contribute to the majority of infant deaths. Signs of premature labor may include a bloody or watery vaginal discharge, pelvic pressure, abdominal cramping, and regular contractions. Women at risk of premature labor include those who:

* are carrying more than one fetus;
* have a history of premature labor or preterm delivery;
* have an abnormally shaped uterus;
* have a history of cervical incompetency;
* use cocaine during pregnancy;

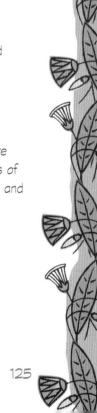

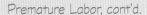

Premature Labor, cont'd.

- have a kidney infection during pregnancy;
- have been exposed to DES in utero;
- have had surgery on their cervix; or
- have too much fluid in the amniotic sac, a condition called "hydramnios."

If there is a possibility of premature labor, you will be watched very closely. Your health-care provider will perform frequent pelvic exams to assess cervical changes. Cervical changes can also be monitored via sonograms. You should refrain from intercourse if there is any sign of premature labor, and immediately call your health-care provider.

## Premature Rupture of Membranes (PROM)

Premature rupture of membranes occurs when leakage of amniotic fluid occurs at least one hour before the onset of labor. It is still safe to deliver within 24 hours and avoid risk of infection. If membranes rupture before the 36th week of gestation, you will be admitted to the hospital to be monitored where your medical team will attempt to delay your delivery until it is safe for the baby. After the membranes rupture, 90 percent of women go into spontaneous labor within 12 to 24 hours. Also see *Water Breaks*.

## Prenatal

The time prior to giving birth.

126

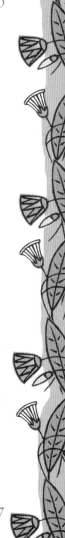

## Prenatal Care

Many studies have demonstrated that the earlier you start prenatal care, the better your pregnancy outcome. As soon as you have missed your first period, you should confirm your pregnancy with your health-care provider. Urine pregnancy tests are very sensitive, and if you are pregnant, you could test positive even before your expected menstrual period. The prenatal medical care you receive gives your health-care provider the opportunity to recognize developing problems and provide treatment.

## Prenatal Visits

The first prenatal visit is usually scheduled by the sixth to tenth week of pregnancy. At the first visit, your health-care provider will take a menstrual history, including the date of your last menstrual period (referred to as the LMP), and note whether this period was normal or abnormal. Your provider will also examine you physically and provide an estimated date of confinement (EDC), which may be confirmed by a sonogram.

Other information that your provider needs to evaluate includes the state of your pregnancy, any drugs you may have taken, and whether you have had any infection or bleeding since the LMP. If you have had other pregnancies, you will be asked if they were at term, premature, or postterm; the progress of the labor; and whether the delivery was vaginal or cesarean. If you had a cesarean section, your provider will want to know the type of incision used on the uterus. For a previous vaginal delivery, you should know which types of instruments, if any, were used, whether the delivery was spontaneous, and if any anesthesia was used. You will also be asked whether there were complications during labor or afterward.

Your family's medical history is also important. How is the health of any living children? What kinds of diseases have you had? What medicines or drugs have you taken? Do you smoke, or did you in the past?

Do you have any allergies? Have you had blood transfusions? What type of birth control did you use prior to the pregnancy? Have you had any pelvic surgeries or any traumas to the pelvis? You should also tell your provider about any hereditary diseases in your and your husband's families. You will also be asked about your employment to determine if it might affect the pregnancy in any way.

Up through the 28th week, you will see your health-care provider every four weeks. After that point and through your 36th week, you will see your provider every two weeks; after the 36th week, you will see your provider weekly until you deliver. Of course, if problems arise, you should be able to see your health-care provider at any time. Your gestational age is determined during each visit. Your urine is tested for sugar and protein; the presence of sugar could signal the possibility of diabetes, and protein could indicate toxemia. Fundal height is measured, as well as your weight, and the fetal heart tone is heard. Other timely tests will also be performed.

## Preterm Labor

When labor begins before the 37th week of gestation, it is considered preterm. It can be treated with bed rest, or hospitalization with intravenous medications to stop your labor. Preterm labor is more common with multiple pregnancies, among women with uterine fibroids or a benign tumor of the uterus, and in cases of cervical incompetency.

## Primapara

A woman having her first baby.

## Progesterone

Progesterone is the female sex hormone that is secreted by the ovaries and adrenal cortex, and is responsible for the preparation of the uterus for receiving the fertilized egg.

## Prolapse Cord

When the umbilical cord descends out of the birth canal before the baby, the cord has prolapsed. This is a rare event. Since the baby's oxygen supply is affected, an emergency cesarean section will have to be performed.

## Prolonged Labor

When labor lasts longer than usual, or progresses very slowly, contractions may need to be speeded with pitocin, or your baby may need to be delivered by cesarean section.

## Protein

During each prenatal visit, your urine is tested for protein. The presence of protein could be a sign of pre-eclampsia.

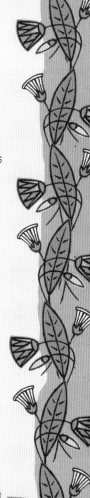

## Pubis or Pubic Area

The frontal bony structure of your pelvis.

## Pushing

When your cervix is fully dilated during labor, you will be instructed to start pushing. If you had an epidural block, you may not be able to feel which muscles to use. Pushing can last from 30 minutes to three hours for your first baby, and from 30 minutes to one hour for subsequent births. You may feel some urge to push toward the end of the first stage of labor, before your cervix has been fully dilated. In this case, you will be asked not to push in order to avoid the swelling of your cervix, which would make it more difficult to dilate. Pushing can be a very exhausting task, but hang in there, for you are almost at the end of the road. You will not believe how strong you are; with some effort, you will find the strength to continue.

## Quickening

Quickening is the perception of the fetus moving inside the uterus. It typically occurs between the 16th and 20th week of pregnancy.

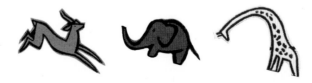

130

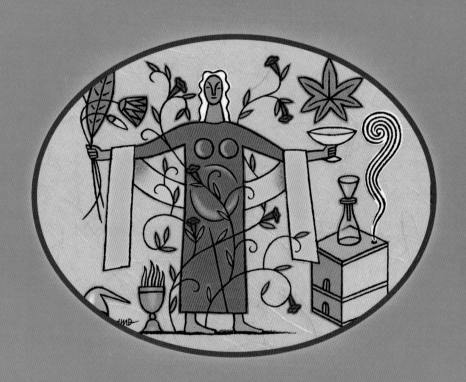

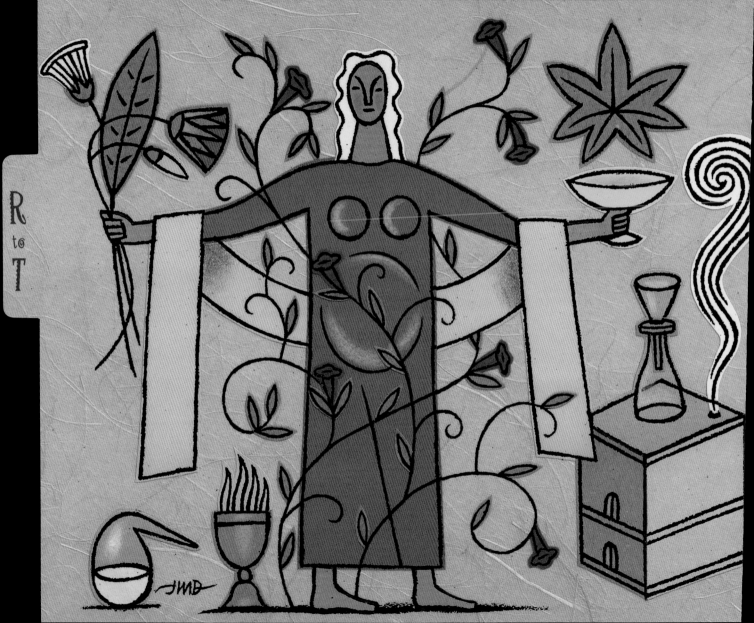

## Rectum

Your rectum is located at the lower end of your colon, ending with your anus, or exit point, from the body.

## Reflexology

Reflexology involves manipulation of specific areas of the feet that correspond to particular organs or body systems that can bring the body into balance. This therapy can be a good way to relax and relieve stress and tension during pregnancy; and can improve circulation among women with varicose veins, hemorrhoids, and swelling.

## Relaxation Techniques

Natural relaxation techniques, such as breathing, meditation, yoga, aromatherapy, massage, acupressure, acupuncture, guided imagery, and self-hypnosis can be used during pregnancy and labor to relieve stress and alleviate pain.

## Retained Placenta

When the placenta fails to separate and is not delivered within 30 minutes after childbirth, your body has retained the placenta. To resolve this problem, your birth attendant will press down on your abdomen while pulling gently on the umbilical cord. Infrequently, the placenta may have to be manually removed.

## Retarded Fetal Growth

Retarded fetal growth occurs when the placenta does not supply enough nourishment to the fetus. This condition may be caused by severe pre-eclampsia, hypertension, bleeding during pregnancy, heart disease, or diabetes.

## Rh Disease

The Rh factor is an antigen, a protein found on the surface of blood cells, which causes an immune response. When an individual lacks the Rh factor, he or she is Rh-negative, and those who have it are Rh-positive. About 15 percent of women are Rh negative. Rh disease or sensitization occurs when an Rh-negative woman, with a partner who is Rh-positive, carries a fetus who is Rh-positive. If the fetus's blood enters her bloodstream, she may develop antibodies that will try to reject the baby's blood, but usually not enough to cause harm during a first pregnancy.

The next time this woman carries another Rh-positive fetus, these antibodies can attack the fetus's red blood cells, causing anemia, organ damage, or even death. Sensitization is prevented by giving the woman a blood product called D (Rho[D]) immune globulin. This is recommended at 28 weeks for the Rh-negative mother who is not sensitized, unless the father is Rh-negative. At birth, if the baby is Rh-positive, another immune globulin inoculation is given to the mother within the first 48 hours after childbirth. D (Rho[D]) immune globulin is also given with any intervention that can result in fetal to maternal bleeding. It is given after an ectopic pregnancy, abortion (spontaneous or induced), CVS sampling, amniocentesis, abdominal trauma, and placental abruption.

## Ripe

A term used to describe the condition of the cervix when ready for the onset of labor.

## Round Ligament Pain

Round ligaments are supporting tissue that stretch from the sides of the uterus to the groin. Round ligament pain is common during the second and third trimester, and consists of sharp pains in the lower abdomen, radiating to one side, and exacerbated by motion. These pains are caused by the stretching of the round ligaments, and they are usually more pronounced on the right side. Self-help treatment includes application of a hot water bottle or heating pad. Avoid sudden movements or standing or sitting too quickly; analgesics are seldom necessary.

## Rubella

Rubella, or German measles, is a common childhood viral disease. If it occurs while a woman is pregnant, it can cause birth defects. During your first prenatal visit, a blood test will be performed to determine if you are immune to rubella. If not, you will receive a rubella vaccine prior to discharge, after the birth of your child. Your immunity to rubella should be checked before you attempt to conceive. If you are not immune, you will receive the vaccine and be instructed to continue with your contraception method for at least three months before trying to conceive.

## Rupture of the Membranes

Rupture of the membranes is what happens when your "water breaks." It usually occurs near term but can be an indication of premature labor. You should immediately report this to your health-care provider; meanwhile, avoid intercourse.

## Seat Belts

It is now required by law that you wear seat belts while riding in an automobile in many states. You should continue to wear your seat belt while driving during your pregnancy. Position the upper part of the belt between your breasts and the lap belt under your abdomen and against your upper thighs.

## Seeing Spots

If you begin to see spots before your eyes during your pregnancy, you should see your health-care provider immediately. This symptom has been associated with pre-eclampsia.

## Sex

This is the term that can either be used to mean the gender of your baby or the act you indulged in to create your baby.

## Sexual Intercourse

Sexual intercourse is the act in which a man places his erect penis into a woman's vagina, also known as making love, sex, and coitus. You can have sexual intercourse throughout pregnancy unless you have a history of premature labor, abnormal bleeding, or a broken amniotic sac (rupture of the membranes). Sexual intercourse will not hurt the baby. Some partners find that a woman is even sexier while pregnant. It is recommended that you wait at least six weeks after the birth of your child before resuming sexual intercourse. Otherwise, you should use an appropriate birth control method.

## Sexually Transmitted Diseases (STDs)

During your first prenatal visit, you will automatically be tested for chlamydia, syphilis, hepatitis B, and gonorrhea. HIV testing is also recommended during pregnancy. STDs, or specific viruses or bacteria, are spread when a person comes in contact with semen, vaginal discharge, or blood of an infected person. A pregnant woman can transmit an STD to her unborn child. Most STDs can be prevented by changing lifestyles, principally through abstinence or with monogamous relationships, and avoiding sexual contact with people who have genital sores or high-risk lifestyles.

## Shortness of Breath

Shortness of breath is a common complaint that occurs in approximately 60 to 70 percent of pregnant women, usually beginning late in the first trimester or early in the second one. Shortness of breath does improve after lightening, when "the baby drops."

## Show

A reddish-colored mucus that occurs at the onset of labor or is gradually discharged during labor.

## SIDS (Sudden Infant Death Syndrome)

SIDS, also called crib death, is the unexplained death of healthy infants while they sleep. The cause is unknown. A variety of explanations have been suggested, but none is completely satisfactory. SIDS has been associated with the baby sleeping on its stomach, women who smoke during pregnancy, and prematurity. SIDS is more common in winter, and it affects boys more than girls.

## Sitz Bath

Sitz baths are a natural remedy in which the pelvis is immersed in warm or cold water. At home, fill your bathtub with water to a level that reaches your navel; at the hospital, after childbirth, a special bowl can be provided for your use.

## Skin Changes

Many skin changes can occur during your pregnancy, primarily due to the increase in hormone levels. You may experience excessive pigmentation, including freckles and darkening of the breast areola. Moles may darken, or your palms may become red, a condition known as palmar erythema. You may notice the formation or worsening of skin tags, or excessive skin growth. By the third trimester, a vertical line appears, leading from the umbilicus to the pubic bone; this line is known as the linea nigra. Occasionally, women experience mysterious red blotches on the abdomen, thighs, arms, or buttocks during the second half of their pregnancy. These blotches may be due to fetal cells migrating to the mother's skin.

## Sleepiness

Another common symptom you may experience during your first trimester of pregnancy is sleepiness. During pregnancy, there is a large increase in the amount of progesterone, which has a sedating effect.

## Smoking

A woman and her partner should stop smoking even before trying to conceive. Nicotine consumption negatively affects male and female fertility and may increase the risk of ectopic pregnancy. Carcinogenic substances found in cigarette smoke may cause damage to the sperm of male smokers and adversely affect the fetus. When a pregnant woman smokes, her growing baby is also smoking. The woman is at an increased risk of having an ectopic pregnancy (where the fetus grows outside the uterus), spontaneous abortion during the first 12 weeks of pregnancy (a miscarriage), and placental abruption (detachment of the placenta, or afterbirth, from the uterine wall). The risks to the baby are low birth weight, a low IQ, greater-than-normal chance of having upper respiratory infections during childhood, cancer, and SIDS (sudden infant death syndrome). Also beware of secondhand smoke; it has the same effects.

## Sonogram

A sonogram, or ultrasound, is a diagnostic technique that uses sound waves to produce images of internal body conditions, such as the health of an unborn child, or a diagnosis of a breast or ovarian cyst. During pregnancy, this test helps the health-care provider examine the baby's internal and external features. It also shows the fetus's position, age, weight, placental site, expected date of delivery, presentation, amount of amniotic fluid, and sometimes the sex. During the first 12 weeks of pregnancy, a vaginal ultrasound is typically performed by inserting a wandlike transducer into your vagina, providing the best possible image of your baby. A sonogram can also help detect causes of bleeding, detect the viability of the fetus, and rule out an ectopic pregnancy, and it is sometimes used to follow women who are at risk. A sonogram is most accurate when performed before the 20th week of pregnancy.

Being able to see your unborn child in your uterus is one of the most exhilarating experiences you'll have during your pregnancy. Proud parents and grandparents now carry sonogram pictures of their unborn babies in their wallets.

## Sound Therapy

Certain sounds have been found to influence brainwave frequency, slow breathing, calm a racing heart, and stimulate mental lucidity. They can also decrease the need for anesthesia and reduce muscle tension, high blood pressure, pain, and physical discomfort. Relaxing music can be played to the baby while in utero. Also, during labor and delivery, music has been demonstrated to enhance comfort, security, and personal control over what is happening in the labor room.

## Sperm

The ejaculate from the male is called sperm. There are about 150 to 350 million sperm in an average ejaculation, but only one tenacious sperm will penetrate the egg's tough outer membrane when they meet in the Fallopian tube. The average life span of sperm is one to three days. (The herb St. John's wort has been found to cause damage to sperm cells.)

## Spotting

The spotting of small amounts of blood may occur at any time during your pregnancy and may be the sign of something wrong. You need to be evaluated by your health-care provider. Spotting is a common sign of miscarriage and ectopic pregnancy.

## Squatting

Squatting is a position to use when pushing during labor, as it increases the size of the vaginal opening.

## Stillbirth

Stillbirth is the birth of a dead baby after the 28th week of pregnancy. About one-third of all stillbirths have no known cause, and they are more common among older women and women with uncontrolled diabetes. The loss of a pregnancy at any stage can be devastating to a woman and her family, causing profound distress. Participation in a support group with other women who have had a similar experience, or one-on-one counseling, can be helpful during this time.

## Stress

Many life events, both positive and negative, can precipitate stress, and pregnancy is no exception. To relieve stress, try the following:

* Exercise regularly. Healthy women with a normal pregnancy can continue with their routine exercise.

* Relaxation techniques such as meditation, progressive muscle relaxation, stretching, guided visual imagery, biofeedback, yoga, and prayer can help. Also, you might find a lukewarm bubble bath to be a great stress reducer.

* Listen to relaxing music.

* Get a massage.

* When we're stressed, we tend to take quick, shallow breaths. To reduce stress, take slow, deep breaths; inhale deeply, filling the entire diaphragm, and hold for a few seconds, then release the air very gradually from your mouth.

## Stress Test

During a stress test, contractions are induced with an intravenous solution called pitocin, which is similar to the natural hormone called oxytocin. Contractions can also be achieved by rubbing your nipples to prompt the release of oxytocin. The fetus's heart rate response to contractions is observed.

## Stretch Marks

Stretch marks are one of the most unwelcome skin changes that result in up to 50 percent of pregnancies. These marks usually appear on the breasts and abdomen and are due to the expansion of your skin. Sorry, there is no way to prevent them. Some creams that are currently being touted to prevent stretch marks only soothe the discomfort caused by the stretching. Stretch marks usually lighten after birth.

## Swelling

Puffiness of the face, hands, and lower extremities is common during pregnancy. Extreme cases may be associated with pre-eclampsia. Massage and reflexology can be utilized to increase circulation. Avoid salty food. If your legs are swollen, avoid standing for long periods of time.

## Syphilis

This sexually transmitted disease, caused by a spiral bacteria called treponema pallidum, is transmitted by direct contact and is characterized by painless sores on the penis and in the vagina, anus, and sometimes in the mouth and throat. Syphilis can be cured with antibiotics. Symptoms usually appear three to four weeks after initial contact. Lesions disappear within five weeks, even without treatment, but the disease itself does not go away if left untreated. Infected women can pass the disease to their unborn children, called congenital syphilis. Infected women also experience a high incidence of spontaneous abortion and stillbirth.

## Tests

Laboratory testing will be performed routinely throughout your prenatal period as appropriate:

* Determination of immunity to rubella, syphilis screen, antibodies to Hepatitis B surface antigen, HIV, and blood type—during your first visit.
* A complete blood count (CBC)—during your first visit.
* Hemoglobin or hematocrit—at 24 to 28 weeks of pregnancy.
* Urinalysis—during the first visit and whenever indicated.
* Antibody screen for Rh disease—during your first visit, repeated at 28 weeks in unsensitized Rh-negative women.
* Glucose screen—at 24 to 28 weeks.
* Group B strep—at 34 to 36 weeks.

## Toxemia

Toxemia is also known as pre-eclampsia.

## Toxoplasmosis

Toxoplasmosis is a medical condition that can cause birth defects. It is caused by a virus that can be found in raw meat and in the feces of cats. Cook your meat until well done. If you own a cat, wash your hands after handling it, and delegate the cleaning of the litter box to someone else. You don't need to get rid of Garfield or Fluffy—just exercise caution.

## Travel

Traveling in cars and pressurized airplanes need not be given up during your pregnancy, but it is advised that you stay close to home during your final weeks. During any long trip, walk around or change positions every half hour or so. Avoiding prolonged sitting during travel is important because of the increased risk of blood clots. Avoid unpressurized private planes. Wear comfortable shoes and support stockings—and always take a copy of your prenatal records with you.

## Trimester

The first trimester is measured from 1 to 12 weeks, the second trimester from 13 to 28 weeks, and the third trimester from 29 to 40 weeks.

## Triplets

When the pregnancy results in three fetuses, you will have triplets. Triplets are rare, occurring naturally in 1 of only 8,000 pregnancies; however, they are more common these days because the use of advanced reproductive technologies is causing more multiple births.

## Tubal Sterilization

A tubal sterilization is a surgical procedure in which the Fallopian tubes are closed off by cauterizing (burning), cutting, or clamping. This procedure is usually performed within the first 24 hours after a vaginal delivery, at the time of a cesarean section, or at any time between pregnancies. Postpartum sterilization can only be performed by consent prior to labor. Remember that for both men and women, sterilization is a permanent decision and should only be considered if you are *certain* you do not want any more children.

## Twin Pregnancy

Twins occur once in every 90 births. Twins are the result of the parallel development of two eggs that are fertilized by two sperm (fraternal twins), each one in its own placenta. Two out of three twins are fraternal twins. Alternately, a single egg splits shortly after fertilization (identical twins), and the fetuses share one placenta between them. Twins are usually discovered by manual examination when the uterus is growing at a faster rate than the gestational age of the pregnancy, or during a routine sonogram. Twin pregnancies are at a higher risk for anemia, placenta previa, preterm labor, and postpartum hemorrhage.

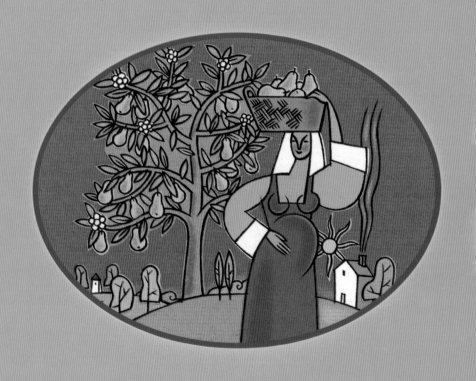

U
to
Z

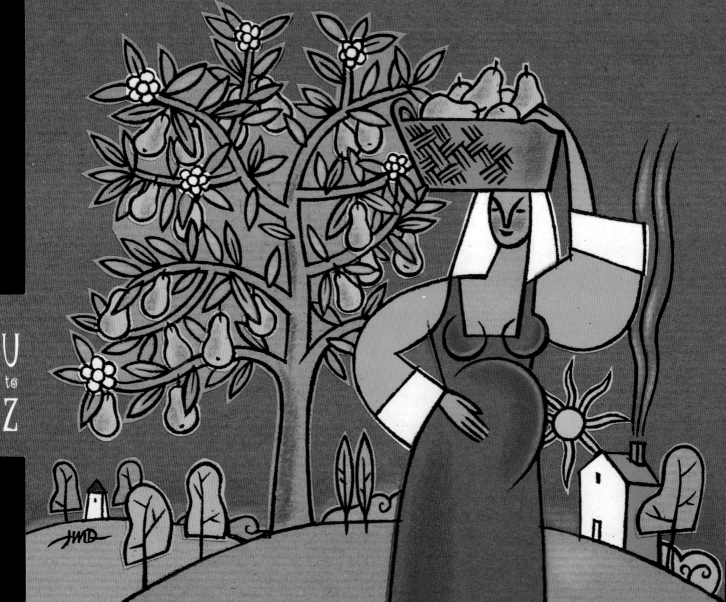

## Ultrasound

Also called a sonogram.

## Umbilical Cord

The umbilical cord consists of one blood vessel to carry oxygenated blood and nutrients to the fetus, and two to carry blood to the placenta for purification and cleansing.

## Umbilicus

The navel or belly button.

## Underwater Birth

An underwater birth is a method of natural childbirth that is thought to ease the birthing transition for the fetus, ease stress and pain for the laboring mother, and lessen the length of labor and difficulty in pushing. Underwater births can be performed at home or in birthing centers. During this type of delivery, a woman enters the water up to her waist after she is fully dilated, then she begins pushing. When the baby is delivered, it is quickly lifted to the mother's breast and allowed to take its first breath.

## Urinary Frequency

Needing to urinate frequently is a common symptom during the first 12 weeks of pregnancy. It recurs near term as the baby's head settles in the pelvis.

## Uterus

The uterus is an inverted, pear-shaped, hollow, muscular organ located in the female pelvic region between the bladder and the rectum. The wider body of the uterus is called the uterine fundus. The uterus provides the necessary environment for a fertilized egg to grow and mature into a baby. The uterus is covered by a smooth outer surface, the perimetrium. Its middle muscular layer is called the myometrium, and the inner lining that is shed each month during menstruation is called the endometrium. During pregnancy, your uterus becomes soft and spherical.

## Vaccine

Any vaccines consisting of live viruses should be avoided during pregnancy. Live vaccines such as oral polio, yellow fever, measles, mumps, or rubella should not be given to pregnant women, or those who are actively trying to conceive. Influenza vaccine should only be given (preferably after the third trimester) to pregnant mothers who have other medical conditions that increase their risk of complications from the flu.

## Vacuum Extraction

During labor, your health-care provider may use a soft plastic or metal cup to pull your baby's head from your vagina. This gadget is attached to a vacuum pump.

## Vagina

The vagina is a three- to four-inch passageway, extending from your uterus to the outside of your body. It functions as the female sexual organ and birth canal. After conception, the number of blood vessels in the vagina increases, giving it a violet hue. The vaginal walls elongate and thicken, becoming loose in preparation for childbirth. The vaginal opening also becomes swollen.

## Vaginal Birth after Cesarean (VBAC)

Having once had a cesarean section (C-section) birth does not necessarily mean that future births will be C-sections. You should discuss your options with your health-care provider. Vaginal births occur in up to 50 to 80 percent of women who previously had a C-section birth.

## Vaginal Discharge

Vaginal discharge is a normal occurrence. Healthy discharge varies throughout your menstrual cycle: usually whitish, but thin and clear around ovulation to facilitate the sperm, and thickening as time progresses until menstruation. During pregnancy, your vaginal discharge remains thick, white, and acidic to help guard against infection. Sometimes, it may be faintly malodorous.

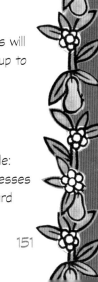

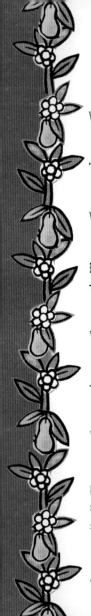

## Vaginal Exam

During labor, you will be checked periodically to evaluate cervical thinning and dilation. The fetus's head "station" will also be determined to tell how far it has progressed into the birth canal.

## Vaginitis

Vaginitis is an inflammation of the vagina, and it is sometimes present without obvious symptoms. Bacterial vaginosis is a bacterial infection that has been associated with preterm labor and can easily be treated with antibiotics. It is associated with a fishy odor and a frothy discharge.

## Variable Deceleration

The fetal heart-rate pattern associated with compression of the umbilical cord during labor is referred to as variable deceleration.

## Varicose Veins

Varicose veins are distended veins in the vagina, thighs, and legs, caused by increased blood volume and pressure in the lower extremities, brought about by the growing uterus. To prevent varicose veins, avoid standing for long periods, don't cross your legs while seated, and try not to wear knee-highs or thigh-high stockings. Rest frequently, and put your feet up whenever possible to improve circulation. Gentle massage increases circulation and is good for varicose veins. If you must stand, lift your heels or toes frequently to promote circulation.

## Venereal Warts

Venereal warts are skin growths that are caused by the human papilloma virus (HPV) and transmitted by sexual contact. Warts of different sizes can show up on, or in, the genital organs and the rectum within six months of initial contact. Sometimes an itching or burning sensation around the genital organs also occurs. Venereal warts do not usually create problems during pregnancy; however, they have a tendency to grow larger in number and size.

## Visual Changes

Contact lenses may become uncomfortable during your pregnancy.

## Vitamins

Only take prenatal vitamins during your pregnancy. An excess of some vitamins may be detrimental to the developing embryo and fetus, causing birth defects.

## Vomiting

Vomiting is a common symptom of early pregnancy. It is often accompanied by nausea and is called "morning sickness." Occasional vomiting is okay. Try to drink lots of fluids so you don't become dehydrated; warm soups and drinks such as Gatorade are preferable. If vomiting increases in intensity, call your health-care provider.

## Vulva

A woman's external genital area is called the vulva, or introitus. During pregnancy, the vulva becomes swollen.

## Water Breaks

Water breaks, also known as the rupture of the "bag of water," may be confused with the passage of urine due to incontinence. Amniotic fluid is usually pale to clear and may include small white chunks, much like cottage cheese. If the fetus has passed meconium, the fluid may be slightly greenish. In any case, call your health-care provider to be checked right away.

## Weight Gain

A woman should gain about 25 pounds during a healthy pregnancy. Approximately 18 pounds is related to the fetus, placenta, amniotic fluid, water retention, and increased blood volume. Pregnancy is not the time to try to lose weight. The average weight loss after childbirth is about 13 pounds, and 3 to 4 more pounds are lost within the first 24 hours. Women who breast-feed their newborn babies lose their pregnancy weight faster than those who don't—yet another benefit of breast-feeding. If you are underweight or overweight before pregnancy, or are carrying multiple fetuses, advice on weight gain differs.

## Work

Some women work until their babies are due, especially if their jobs are sedentary. You should try to take frequent short breaks during your work day. If there are any signs of complications, you should follow your health-care provider's advice. If necessary, stop working and go on disability.

In California, a pregnant woman is entitled to state disability at four weeks before her due date, and from six to eight weeks after delivery. In companies where there are more than 50 workers, the Family Medical Leave Act requires that your employer provide 12 weeks unpaid leave for childbirth. You will need to give a 30-day notice unless you have an emergency.

## Workplace

Environmental hazards encountered at the workplace may decrease fertility and increase the risk of miscarriage, fetal malformation, and preterm delivery. At work, stay away from chemicals, and avoid prolonged standing and lifting of more than 20 pounds. Also avoid x-rays.

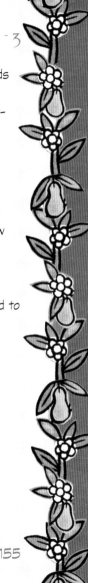

155

## X-ray

Radiation of the body should be limited to emergency cases during pregnancy. It is okay to have dental x-rays, provided you are shielded with a lead apron.

## Yeast

During pregnancy, a woman may be more prone to yeast infections. Avoid tight clothing and wear panty hose with a cotton crotch. Yogurt and acidophilus in your diet can help prevent yeast infections.

## Yoga

Yoga has been used to relieve pregnancy-related stress, hypertension, depression, and diabetes. It is good for pushing because it helps you concentrate on one part of your body at a time. Yoga can also help with breathing during labor, and pain relief.

## Zygote

When the tenacious sperm enters a mature egg and fertilizes it, it is then called a zygote, on the way to becoming a fetus, and then your baby.

# About the Author

CAROLLE JEAN-MURAT, M.D., F.A.C.O.G., is a board-certified obstetrician and gynecologist, and a Fellow of the American College of Obstetricians and Gynecologists. She has had a private practice in San Diego, California, since 1982.

Dr. Carolle was born and raised in Haiti where at 11 years of age she begged her mother to let her help with a home delivery. After graduating from medical school in Mexico, she did a year of internship at Cornwall Regional Hospital in Jamaica, where she learned to do natural deliveries with certified nurse-midwives. She then returned to rural Mexico for a year of community medicine, where she performed deliveries at home, often with no running water or electricity available. Dr. Carolle then came to the United States for postgraduate training in obstetrics and gynecology at Mount Sinai Medical Center in Milwaukee, Wisconsin.

Dr. Carolle is an Assistant Clinical Professor at the University of California at San Diego (UCSD) School of Medicine, Department of Reproductive Endocrinology. She is also a clinical mentor for underserved students at San Diego State University. She is a motivational speaker who brings her message of self-empowerment to women through lectures, TV and radio appearances, a Spanish-language newspaper column, articles, and audiocassettes.

Besides authoring *Menopause Made Easy: How to Make the Right Decisions for the Rest of Your Life*, she wrote the award-winning book, *Staying Healthy: 10 Easy Steps for Women*, available in both English and Spanish. Dr. Carolle is also a contributing author of *Millennium 2000: A Positive Approach*, with Louise L. Hay and Friends.

Dr. Carolle can be reached at www.drcarolle.com

157

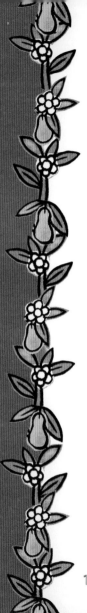

# Hay House Lifestyles Titles

### Flip Books

*101 Ways to Happiness*, by Louise L. Hay

*101 Ways to Health and Healing*, by Louise L. Hay

*101 Ways to Romance*, by Barbara De Angelis, Ph.D.

*101 Ways to Transform Your Life*,
by Dr. Wayne W. Dyer

### Books

*A Garden of Thoughts*, by Louise L. Hay

*Aromatherapy A-Z*, by Connie Higley, Alan Higley,
and Pat Leatham

*Aromatherapy 101*, by Karen Downes

*Colors & Numbers*, by Louise L. Hay

*Constant Craving A-Z*, by Doreen Virtue, Ph.D.

*Dream Journal*, by Leon Nacson

*Healing with Herbs and Home Remedies A-Z*,
by Hanna Kroeger

*Healing with the Angels Oracle Cards*
(booklet and card pack), by Doreen Virtue, Ph.D.

*Heal Your Body A-Z*, by Louise L. Hay

*Home Design with Feng Shui A-Z*,
by Terah Kathryn Collins

*Homeopathy A-Z*, by Dana Ullman, M.P.H.

*Interpreting Dreams A-Z*, by Leon Nacson

*Natural Gardening A-Z*, by Donald W. Trotter, Ph.D.

*Natural Pregnancy A-Z*, by Carolle Jean-Murat, M.D.

*Pleasant Dreams*, by Amy E. Dean

*Weddings A-Z*, by Deborah McCoy

*What Color Is Your Personality?*
by Carol Ritberger, Ph.D.

*What Is Spirit?*, by Lexie Brockway Potamkin

*You Can Heal Your Life*, by Louise L. Hay . . . and

*Power Thought Cards*, by Louise L. Hay
(affirmation cards)

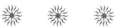

All of the above titles may be ordered by calling
Hay House at the numbers on the next page.

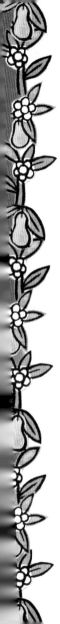
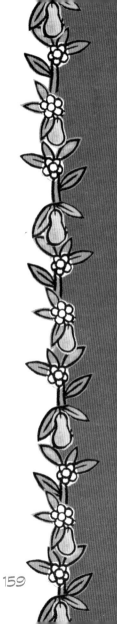

We hope you enjoyed
this Hay House Lifestyles book.
If you would like to receive a free catalog featuring additional
Hay House books and products, or if you would like information about the
Hay Foundation, please contact:

Hay House, Inc.
P.O. Box 5100
Carlsbad, CA 92018-5100

(760) 431-7695 or (800) 654-5126
(760) 431-6948 (fax) or (800) 650-5115 (fax)

Please visit the Hay House Website at: www.hayhouse.com

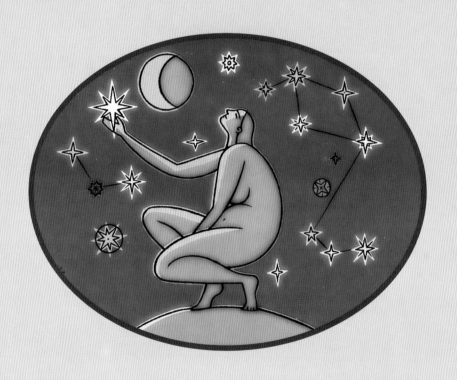